Clinical Anatomy
for Your Pocket

Douglas J. Gould, Ph.D.

Associate Professor, Division of Anatomy
The Ohio State University College of Medicine
Columbus, Ohio

D0968012

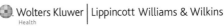

Wolters Kluwer | Lippincott Williams & Wilkins
Health

Philadelphia · Baltimore · New York · London
Buenos Aires · Hong Kong · Sydney · Tokyo

Acquisitions Editor: Crystal Taylor
Managing Editor: Kelly Horvath
Marketing Manager: Jennifer Kuklinski

Production Editor: Beth Martz
Design Coordinator: Stephen Druding
Compositor: Aptara®

351 West Camden Street
Baltimore, MD 21201

530 Walnut Street
Philadelphia, PA 19106

Printed in the People's Republic of China

9 8 7 6 5 4 3 2 1

Library of Congress Cataloging-in-Publication Data

Gould, Douglas J.
  Clinical anatomy for your pocket / Douglas J. Gould.
      p. ; cm.
  Includes index.
  ISBN-13: 978-0-7817-9193-9 (pbk. : alk. paper)
  ISBN-10: 0-7817-9193-6 (pbk. : alk. paper) 1. Human anatomy—
Outlines, syllabi, etc. I. Title.
  [DNLM: 1. Anatomy. QS 4 G696c 2009]
  QM31.G68 2009
  611—dc22

                                                    2008024080

DISCLAIMER

To purchase additional copies of this book, call our customer service department at **(800) 638-3030** or fax orders to **(301) 223-2320**. International customers should call **(301) 223-2300**.

Visit Lippincott Williams & Wilkins on the Internet: http://www.lww.com. Lippincott Williams & Wilkins customer service representatives are available from 8:30 am to 6:00 pm, EST.

Health professions' curricula around the world are continually evolving: new discoveries, techniques, applications, and content areas compete for increasingly limited time with traditional basic science topics such as gross anatomy. It is in this context that the foundations established in gross anatomy become increasingly important and relevant for absorbing and applying our ever-expanding knowledge of the human body. As a result of the progressively more crowded curricular landscape, students and instructors are finding new ways to maximize precious contact, preparation, and study time through more efficient, high-yield presentation and study methods.

Clinical Anatomy for Your Pocket is designed to serve the time-crunched student. The presentation of gross anatomy in bullet and table format streamlines study and exam preparation. This pocket size, quick reference book is portable, practical, and necessary; even at this small size, nothing is omitted and a large number of clinically significant facts, mnemonics, and easy-to-learn concepts are used to complement the tables and inform the reader.

I am confident that *Clinical Anatomy for Your Pocket* will greatly benefit all students attempting to learn clinically relevant anatomy in a variety of settings, including all graduate and professional gross anatomy programs.

Dedication

I dedicate this book to my mother—Margaret.
My first teacher.

Acknowledgments

I would like to thank the student reviewers for their input into this book: I hope that I have done you justice and created the learning tool that you need. I would also like to thank Dr. Robert DePhilip, the faculty reviewer of *Clinical Anatomy for Your Pocket*, whose suggestions have proved invaluable in creating an accurate and functional tool for students.

Contents

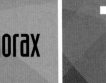

Thorax

INTRODUCTION

The thorax is that portion of the trunk inferior to the neck (superior thoracic aperture) and superior to the diaphragm, to which the pectoral girdle and upper limbs are attached.

THORACIC WALL

The bones of the thoracic wall are the ribs and sternum. Ribs 3–9 possess characteristics common to the majority of ribs and so are considered "typical," whereas ribs 1–2 and 10–12 have specializations or are lacking typical characteristics and so are considered "atypical."

Bones of the thoracic wall

Bone	Characteristic	Significance
Typical ribs (3–9)	Head	Bears 2 facets that articulate with vertebra of same number and the vertebra superior to it
	Neck	Joins head with body of rib
	Tubercle	• Articulates with transverse process of vertebra of same number • Located at junction of neck and body
	Body	• Bears pronounced angle • Inferior internal border has costal groove for intercostal neurovascular elements
Atypical ribs (1–2, 10–12)	• 1st and 2nd ribs—heads • Ribs 10–12 sternal attachments	• The heads of the first 2 ribs only attach to one vertebral body, unlike typical ribs that attach to two • The 1st and 2nd ribs have additional tubercles for muscle attachments

(continued)

Bones of the thoracic wall *(continued)*

Bone	Characteristic	Significance
		• Ribs 10–12 attach indirectly (rib 10) or not at all to the sternum (ribs 11–12, the floating ribs)
Thoracic vertebrae (12)	Body	Supports weight
	Spinous process	Serve for muscle attachments
	Transverse process	
	Laminae and pedicles	Form **vertebral arch** that encloses spinal cord
	Vertebral foramen	• Formed from vertebral arch and posterior aspect of vertebral body • Encloses spinal cord • Successive vertebral foramen form vertebral canal
	Vertebral notches— superior and inferior	Inferior and superior notches of adjacent vertebrae form intervertebral foramen that permits passage of spinal nerves between the vertebral canal and periphery
	Articulating processes— superior (2) and inferior (2)	Form zygapophyseal joints with articulating processes on adjacent vertebrae
Sternum	Manubrium	• Superior part of sternum • Superior border bears jugular notch • Clavicular notches (2) are found on each side of the jugular notch for articulation with the clavicles
	Sternal angle	• Landmark for the 2nd ribs' costal cartilage articulation with the sternum • Marks articulation between manubrium and body
	Body	Bears costal notches along lateral border for articulation with costal cartilages
	Xiphoid process	• Most inferior part of sternum • Landmark for central tendon of diaphragm, superior margin of liver, and inferior border of heart

Additional Concept

True, False, and Floating Ribs

Ribs 1–7 are considered "true" ribs, as they attach to the sternum via their individual costal cartilages; ribs 8–10 are considered "false" ribs, as they attach indirectly to the sternum via the costal cartilages of more superior ribs; ribs 11–12 are considered "floating" ribs, as they do not connect to the sternum.

Clinical Significance

Rib Fracture

Fracture of the upper ribs may injure the lungs and of lower ribs may damage the liver or spleen or may tear the diaphragm. All rib fractures are painful owing to the broken pieces moving during respiration, coughing, sneezing, or laughing.

Sternal Puncture

A wide-bore needle may be used to harvest bone marrow from the sternum for transplantation or biopsy.

Muscles of the thoracic wall

(Figures 1-2 and 1-4)

Muscle	Proximal attachment	Distal Attachment	Innervation	Main Actions
External intercostal	Inferior aspect of ribs	Superior aspect of ribs	Intercostal nerves	Elevate ribs
Internal inter-costal				Depress and elevate ribs
Innermost intercostal				
Transverse thoracic	Posterior inferior aspect of sternum	Posterior aspect of costal cartilages 2–6		Depress ribs
Subcostal	Deep aspect of lower ribs, near angles	Superior aspect of 2–3 ribs below proximal attachment		Depress and elevate ribs

(continued)

Muscles of the thoracic wall *(continued)*

Muscle	Proximal attachment	Distal Attachment	Innervation	Main Actions
Diaphragm	Sternum, inferior 6 ribs and their costal cartilages, medial & lateral arcuate ligaments, and 1st 3 lumbar vertebrae	Central tendon of the diaphragm	Motor: phrenic; sensory: phrenic and intercostal nerves	Increases the volume of the thorax to cause inspiration
Levator costarum	T7–T11 transverse processes	Subjacent ribs between tubercle and angle	C8–T11 posterior rami	Elevate ribs
Serratus posterior superior	Nuchal ligament, C7–T3 spinous processes	2nd–4th ribs superior borders	2nd–5th intercostals	
Serratus posterior inferior	T11–L2 spinous processes	8th–12th ribs inferior borders, near angles	9th–11th intercostals and subcostal	Depress ribs

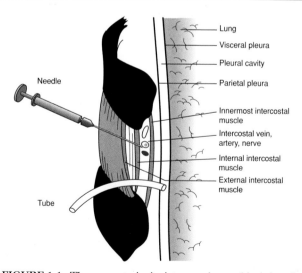

Lung

Visceral pleura

Pleural cavity

Parietal pleura

Needle

Innermost intercostal muscle

Intercostal vein, artery, nerve

Internal intercostal muscle

External intercostal muscle

Tube

FIGURE 1-1. Thoracocentesis. An intercostal nerve block (needle in image) produces anesthesia of an intercostal space by introduction of an anesthetic agent around the intercostal nerve and its collaterals. The tube in the diagram indicates the position for thoracocentesis. (From Dudek RW, Louis TM. *High-Yield Gross Anatomy.* 3rd ed. Baltimore: Lippincott Williams & Wilkins; 2008:56.)

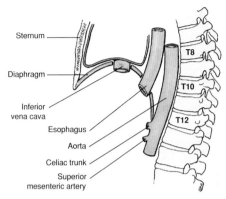

FIGURE 1-2. Holes in diaphragm. There are three large aper- tures in the diaphragm for major structures to pass to and from the thorax into the abdomen. The caval opening for the inferior vena cava (IVC), most anterior, is at the T8 level and to the right of the midline; the esophageal hiatus, intermediate, is at T10 and to the left of the midline; the aortic hiatus for the aorta passes posterior to the vertebral attachment of the diaphragm in the midline at T12. (From Moore KL, Dalley AF. *Clinically Oriented Anatomy.* 5th ed. Baltimore: Lippincott Williams & Wilkins; 2006:329.)

Additional Concept
Diaphragm
The **diaphragm** has three openings that permit passage of structures between the thorax and abdomen. These open- ings are found at T8—caval foramen, T10—esophageal hia- tus, and T12—aortic hiatus.

Clinical Significance
Phrenic Nerve Injury
Phrenic nerve injury results in hemiparalysis of the diaphragm and paradoxical movement during inspiration. Instead of descending during inspiration, the paralyzed half ascends in response to increased intra-abdominal pressure.

Nerves of the thoracic wall

(Figures 1-1 and 1-4)

Nerve	Origin	Structures Innervated
Intercostals	Anterior rami of T1–T11	Intercostal muscles and parietal pleura
Subcostal	Anterior rami of T12	Abdominal wall musculature and parietal pleura
Rami communicantes	Connect intercostals and subcostal nerves to sympathetic trunk	• White—convey presynaptic sympathetic fibers from spinal nerve to sympathetic chain and visceral afferents to spinal nerves • Gray—convey postsynaptic sympathetic fibers from the sympathetic chain to spinal nerve
Sympathetic trunk	Sympathetic chain ganglia (paravertebral ganglia)	Composed of sympathetic ganglia containing postsynaptic sympathetic cell bodies connected by ascending and descending fibers
Thoracic splanchnics	Sympathetic chain: • Greater—T5–T9 • Lesser—T10–T11 • Least—T12	Convey presynaptic sympathetic fibers to the prevertebral ganglia of the abdomen; convey visceral afferents to the sympathetic chain

Arterial supply of the thoracic wall

(Figures 1-1 and 1-4)

Artery	Origin	Description
Internal thoracic	Subclavian	Gives rise to anterior intercostals and musculophrenic
Anterior intercostals	Internal thoracic (1–6) and musculophrenic (7–9)	Supplies intercostal muscles and parietal pleura
Posterior intercostals	Supreme intercostal (1–2) and thoracic aorta	
Subcostal	Thoracic aorta	Supplies anterolateral abdominal musculature

Additional Concept

Venous Drainage

Venous drainage of the thoracic wall generally parallels arterial supply. However, the posterior intercostal veins drain to the azygos system, which is discussed with the posterior mediastinum.

Joints of the thoracic wall

Joint	Type	Articulation	Structure
1st sternocostal	Cartilaginous	1st costal cartilage with manubrium	Joint strengthened by sternocostal radiate ligaments
2nd–7th sternocostal	Synovial	2nd–7th costal cartilages with sternum	
Sternoclavicular	Synovial	Sternal end of clavicle with manubrium and 1st costal cartilage	• Divided into two compartments by articular disc • Joint strengthened by anterior and posterior sternoclavicular and costoclavicular ligaments
Manubriosternal	Cartilaginous	Manubrium with body of sternum	Joint often fuses in older people
Xiphisternal		Xiphoid process with body of sternum	
Interchondral	• 6th–9th: synovial • 9th–10th: fibrous	Costal cartilages of adjacent ribs 6–10	Strengthened by interchondral ligaments
Costochondral	Cartilaginous	Costal cartilage with end of rib	• Bound together by periosteum • Little if any movement permitted
Intervertebral	Symphysis	Adjacent vertebral bodies	Strengthened by anterior and posterior longitudinal ligaments and the anular ligament

(continued)

Joints of the thoracic wall *(continued)*

Joint	Type	Articulation	Structure
Costovertebral	Synovial	Head of ribs with vertebral bodies at same level and the vertebral body superior to it	• Strengthened by radiate and intra-articular ligaments • 1st, 11th, 12th, and and sometimes 10th ribs articulate only with vertebral body of same level
Costotransverse		Tubercle of rib with transverse process of vertebral body at same level	• Strengthened by lateral and superior costotransverse ligaments • 11th and 12th ribs do not participate in costotransverse joints

BREAST

The breast extends from the sternum to the midaxillary line and from ribs 2–6. It rests on the pectoral fascia and the fascia over serratus anterior.

Structure of the breast
(Figure 1-3)

Structure	Description	Significance
Mammary glands	• Modified sweat glands • Arranged in 15–20 lobules	• Accessory reproductive organs in the female • Contained within the breast
Areola	• The skin around the nipple • Studded with sebaceous glands that form elevations	• Turns a darker color during pregnancy • Stimulation from the suckling infant triggers ejection and production of milk—the let-down reflex
Nipple	• Round, raised area of skin in the center of the areola • Surrounded by circularly arranged smooth muscle fibers that cause erection on stimulation	Stimulation from the suckling infant triggers erection of the nipple and the ejection and production of milk

(continued)

Structure of the breast *(continued)*

Structure	Description	Significance
Suspensory ligaments	Connective tissue supports that extend from the dermis to the pectoral fascia	• Provide support for the breast • If invaded by carcinoma, the ligaments shorten and produce skin dimpling and nipple inversion
Lactiferous duct	15–20 total, open onto the nipple	Drain the mammary glandular tissue
Lactiferous sinus	Expansion of lactiferous duct near the nipple	Function as a milk reservoir during lactation
Axillary process	Extension of breast tissue into the axilla	High percentage of breast tumors occurs here

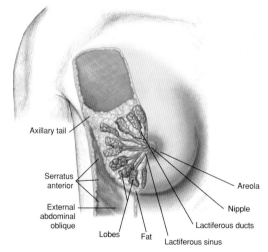

Axillary tail

Serratus anterior

External abdominal oblique

Lobes   Fat   Lactiferous sinus

Areola

Nipple

Lactiferous ducts

FIGURE 1-3. Breast, anterior view. (From Tank PW, Gest TR. *LWW Atlas of Anatomy.* Baltimore: Lippincott Williams & Wilkins; 2009:39.)

Additional Concept

The size and shape of the adult female breast is due to its contained fat, which forms the bulk of the breast tissue.

Clinical Significance

Quadrants

The breast is divided into four **quadrants** for the anatomic location and description of pathologies. The inferior quadrants are less vascular and, therefore, the preferred area for surgical incisions when necessary.

Retromammary Space

Between the breast and the pectoral fascia is the retromammary space, which permits movement of the breast on the thoracic wall. Diminishment of this movement may indicate pathology.

Nerves of the breast

Nerve	Origin	Structures Innervated
Anterior cutaneous branches	Intercostal nerves 4–6	• Sensory to skin of breast • Postsynaptic sympathetic fibers to the smooth muscle of the nipple and blood vessels
Lateral cutaneous branches		

Arterial supply of the breast

Artery	Origin	Description
Medial mammary branches	Internal thoracic	Supplies medial aspect of breast
Anterior intercostals		
Lateral mammary branches	Lateral thoracic	Supplies lateral aspect of breast
Thoracoacromial	Axillary	Supplies breast through pectoral branches
Posterior intercostals	Thoracic aorta	Supplies lateral aspect of breast through lateral mammary branches

Additional Concept

Venous drainage of the breast parallels the arterial supply and drains mainly to the axillary vein, whereas some venous drainage is to the internal thoracic vein.

Lymphatics of the breast

Knowledge of the lymphatic drainage of the breast is important owing to the high incidence of breast carcinoma.

Lymphatic Structure	Description	Drainage
Subareolar lymphatic plexus	Located deep to the nipple, areola, and around the lobules of the glandular tissue of the breast	Drains lymph from the nipple, areola, and glandular tissue of the breast to regional nodes
Axillary lymph nodes	Composed of pectoral, humeral, subscapular, central, and apical nodes	Drains ~75% of lymph from the breast—the lateral quadrant in particular
Parasternal lymph nodes	Located along the sternum	Drains mostly lymph from the medial quadrant of the breast
Abdominal lymph nodes	Located inferior to the diaphragm in the abdominal cavity; also known as inferior phrenic lymph nodes	Drains mostly lymph from the inferior quadrants of the breast
Infraclavicular lymph nodes	Located inferior to the clavicle	Drains lymph from the axillary lymph nodes
Supraclavicular lymph nodes	Located superior to the clavicle	
Subclavian lymphatic trunk	Formed from efferent vessels of the axillary nodes, apical in particular	• On the right—joins with bronchomediastinal & jugular trunks to form the **right lymphatic duct** • On the left—joins the **thoracic duct**

Additional Concept

The contralateral breast receives a significant amount of lymphatic drainage.

MISCELLANEOUS

Thoracic cavity

The thoracic cavity is bounded by the thoracic wall—a flexible musculoskeletal cage. It is divided into 2 laterally placed pleural cavities and a central region—the mediastinum. The thoracic cavity contains the heart, lungs, thymus, trachea, esophagus, and multiple neurovascular elements.

Area	Structure	Significance
Superior thoracic aperture	Boundaries: • Anterior—manubrium • Posterior—T1 • Lateral—1st ribs and their costal cartilages	• Also known as the thoracic inlet • Allows passage of the trachea, esophagus, and neurovascular elements between the thoracic cavity and the neck
Inferior thoracic aperture	Boundaries: • Anterior—xiphisternal joint • Anterolateral—costal cartilages of ribs 7–10—the costal margin • Posterior—T12 • Posterolateral—11th and 12th ribs	• Also known as the thoracic outlet • Closed by the diaphragm • Allows for passage of the inferior vena cava, aorta, and esophagus between the thoracic cavity and abdomen
Intercostal space	Space between adjacent ribs and costal cartilages	Contains intercostal muscles and intercostal neurovascular elements
Superior mediastinum	• Superior border—superior thoracic aperture • Inferior border—plane passing from sternal angle through the T4–T5 vertebral level • Lateral borders—pleural cavities	Contains superior vena cava, brachiocephalic veins, arch of aorta, thoracic duct, esophagus, trachea, left & right vagus nerves, left recurrent laryngeal nerve and left & right phrenic nerves, and the thymus
Inferior mediastinum	• Superior border—plane passing from sternal angle through the T4–T5 vertebral level • Inferior border—diaphragm • Lateral borders—pleural cavities	Subdivided by the pericardial sac into anterior, middle, and posterior mediastina
Anterior mediastinum	• Most anterior part of the inferior mediastinum • Bounded anteriorly by the sternum and transverse thoracic muscle and posteriorly by the pericardium	Contains the thymus, loose connective tissue, sternopericardial ligaments, lymph nodes, and fat
Middle mediastinum	Middle part of inferior mediastinum	Contains the heart, pericardial sac, roots of the great vessels, arch of the azygos vein, and primary bronchi
Posterior mediastinum	Most posterior part of the inferior mediastinum	Contains the thoracic aorta, esophagus, azygos and hemiazygos veins, vagus nerves, thoracic duct, sympathetic trunks, and splanchnic nerves

Mnemonic

V-A-N: Intercostal neurovascular elements are arranged from superior to inferior as:

intercostal **V**ein
intercostal **A**rtery
intercostal **N**erve

Clinical Significance

Thoracic Outlet Syndrome

Obstructions in the root of the neck may affect structures passing through the superior thoracic aperture; problems are often manifested in the upper limb.

Posterior mediastinum

Structure	Significance
Organ	
Esophagus	• Located posterior to the trachea, anterior to vertebral bodies • Begins at inferior aspect of pharynx (C6) • Terminates by entering the stomach after passing through the esophageal hiatus (T10) of the diaphragm
Nerve	
Esophageal plexus	• Formed of parasympathetic fibers from the vagus nerves and sympathetic fibers from sympathetic chain ganglia and the greater splanchnic nerve • Supply glands and musculature of inferior 2/3 of esophagus
Sympathetic trunks	• Located on either side of the vertebral column along posterior wall of the thorax • Chain of paravertebral ganglia containing presynaptic sympathetic cell bodies • Ganglia connected by presynaptic sympathetic and visceral afferent fibers • Connected to thoracic spinal nerves by rami communicantes
Thoracic splanchnic nerves	• Greater, lesser, and least • Convey presynaptic sympathetic fibers from T5–T12 to prevertebral ganglia of the abdomen • Convey visceral afferents from the abdomen
Vessel	
Thoracic aorta	• Continuation of the arch of the aorta; becomes abdominal aorta after passing through the aortic hiatus (T12) of the diaphragm • Found to the left of thoracic vertebral bodies

(continued)

Posterior mediastinum *(continued)*

Structure	Significance
Bronchial arteries	• Left: branches of thoracic aorta • Right: branches of posterior intercostal arteries • Supply oxygenated blood to the tissues of the lung
Pericardial arteries	• Branches of thoracic aorta and pericardiophrenic arteries • Supply the pericardium
Posterior intercostal arteries—9 pairs	• Branches of thoracic aorta • Supply intercostal spaces 3–11
Superior phrenic arteries	• Branches of the thoracic aorta • Supply the diaphragm
Esophageal arteries	• Branches of the thoracic aorta • Supply the esophagus
Subcostal arteries	• Branches of the thoracic aorta • Supply body wall inferior to the 12th ribs
Thoracic duct	• Conveys lymph from entire body, except the right upper limb, right aspect of the thorax and right side of head & neck • Begins in abdomen at chyle cistern and empties into the junction of left internal jugular vein and left subclavian vein • Found along the vertebral column between the azygos vein and esophagus
Azygos vein	• Drains mediastinum and posterior thoracic & abdominal walls on the right; found on right side of vertebral bodies • Begins in the abdomen and terminates by emptying into superior vena cava • Receives hemiazygos and accessory hemiazygos veins at the T8–T9 vertebral level
Hemiazygos vein	• Drains mediastinum and posterior thoracic and abdominal walls on the left as high as T9 vertebral level, where it crosses to the right side to enter the azygos vein
Accessory hemiazygos vein	• Drains mediastinum and posterior upper thoracic wall on the left as far inferiorly as T8 vertebral level where it crosses to the right side to enter the azygos vein

The trachea is presented with the superior mediastinum.

Clinical Significance

Esophageal Constrictions

Three constrictions of the esophagus occur where it is compressed by, from superior to inferior: (1) arch of the aorta, (2) left main bronchus, and (3) the diaphragm. These constrictions are areas susceptible to damage from swallowing caustic substances and are places where ingested objects

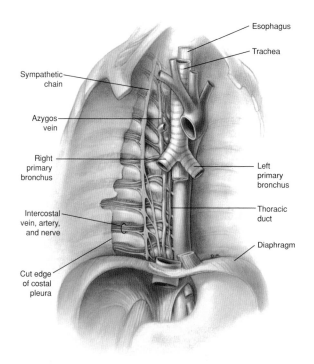

FIGURE 1-4. Posterior mediastinum viewed from the right: parietal pleura is intact on left side and partially removed on right. A portion of esophagus, between bifurcation of trachea and diaphragm, is also removed. (From Agur AMR, Dalley AF. *Grant's Atlas of Anatomy*, 12th ed. Baltimore: Lippincott Williams & Wilkins; 2009:82.)

may become lodged; the constrictions are visible on radiographs and are useful landmarks.

Azygos Veins

The **azygos system** provides a collateral pathway for venous blood that connects the superior and inferior vena cavae.

Mnemonic

Four birds of the thorax:

esopha**GOOSE**
va**GOOSE** nerve
azy**GOOSE** vein
thoracic **DUCK**

Superior mediastinum
(Figure 1-5)

Structure	Significance
Ligamentum arteriosum	• Remnant of the ductus arteriosus (shunt for blood from the fetal pulmonary trunk to aorta) • Connects left pulmonary artery to the arch of the aorta • Left recurrent laryngeal nerve wraps around to then ascend to the larynx
Organ	
Thymus	• Located mostly in the superior mediastinum • Lymphatic organ that involutes after puberty and is replaced by fat
Trachea	• Located anterior to the esophagus • Begins at cricoid cartilage of the larynx • Terminates at the level of the sternal angle into 2 main bronchi • Skeleton of posteriorly oriented U-shaped rings, posterior deficiency spanned by the trachealis muscle
Esophagus	• Located posterior to the trachea and anterior to the vertebral bodies • Begins at inferior aspect of the pharynx, terminates by entering the stomach after passing through the esophageal hiatus (T10) of the diaphragm
Nerve	
Left vagus	• Found anterior to the arch of the aorta where it gives off the left recurrent laryngeal nerve • Passes posterior to the root of the lung, where it ramifies to contribute to the pulmonary, cardiac, and esophageal plexuses
Right vagus	• Found anterior to the right subclavian artery, where it gives off the right recurrent laryngeal nerve • Passes posterior to the root of the lung, where it ramifies to contribute to the pulmonary, cardiac, and esophageal plexuses
Left recurrent laryngeal	• Branch of left vagus nerve as it passes over the anterior surface of the arch of the aorta • Ascends to the larynx between the trachea and esophagus
Right recurrent laryngeal	• Branch of the right vagus nerve as it passes over the anterior surface of the right subclavian artery • Ascends to the larynx between the trachea and esophagus in the tracheoesophageal groove
Left phrenic nerve	• Passes anterior to the root of the lung, found between the fibrous pericardium and mediastinal pleura
Right phrenic nerve	• Sole motor supply to the diaphragm • Sensory to central aspects of diaphragm

(continued)

Superior mediastinum *(continued)*

Structure	Significance
Vessel	
Left brachioce-phalic vein	• Formed by junction of the internal jugular and subclavian veins • The left and right brachiocephalic veins join to form the superior vena cava
Right brachioce-phalic vein	
Superior vena cava	Drains most venous blood from structures superior to the thorax into the right atrium

Arch of the aorta	• Continuation of the ascending aorta; becomes the thoracic aorta as it descends
	• Gives off 3 branches in the superior mediastinum:
	  1. brachiocephalic trunk
	  2. left common carotid artery
	  3. left subclavian artery
	• Left vagus nerve courses on its anterior surface

Brachioce-phalic trunk	• 1st branch of the arch of the aorta • Terminates by dividing into the right common carotid and right subclavian arteries • Indirectly supplies the right side of head and neck and right upper limb through its branches
Left common carotid artery	• 2nd branch of the arch of the aorta • Terminates in the neck by dividing into internal & external carotid arteries • Indirectly supplies left side of head and neck through its branches
Left sub-clavian artery	• 3rd branch of the arch of the aorta • Continues as it passes over the lateral border of the 1st rib to become the left axillary artery • Supplies the left upper limb

The thoracic duct is presented with the posterior mediastinum.

Additional Concept

Lymphatic Drainage

In addition to the brachiocephalic veins forming at the junction of the internal jugular and subclavian veins, it is also the point where the **right lymphatic duct** joins the venous system on the right and the **thoracic** duct on the left—known as the **jugular angle**.

Structure of the pericardial cavity
(Figure 1-5)

Structure	Description	Significance
Pericardial sac	Formed of 2 layers: 1. outer—fibrous pericardium 2. inner—parietal layer of serous pericardium	• Double-layered fibroserous sac that encloses the heart • Fused with adventitia of the great vessels • Attached to the deep surface of the sternum by the sterno-pericardial ligament • Fuses with the central tendon of the diaphragm; therefore, moves during respiration
Visceral layer of serous pericardium	Mesothelium—simple squamous epithelium	Also known as the epicardium—the outer layer of the heart
Parietal layer of serous pericardium		Lines inner surface of fibrous pericardium
Pericardial cavity	Potential space between the layers of serous pericardium	• Filled with serous fluid • Allows heart to beat in a friction free environment
Fibrous pericardium	• Strong collagenous outer layer of the pericardial sac • Fuses with adventitia of great vessels, central tendon of the diaphragm, and sternum	• Inflexible nature prevents overfilling of the heart • Phrenic nerve travels inferiorly through the thorax on its lateral surface
Transverse sinus	Extension of the pericardial cavity posterior to the pulmonary trunk and aorta	Allows for control of blood out of the heart during surgery
Oblique sinus	Extension of the pericardial cavity on the posterior aspect of the heart	Ends as a cul-de-sac between the pulmonary veins

MEDIASTINUM

Additional Concept

Pericardium

The pericardium receives its arterial supply from the pericardiacophrenic arteries, which run with the phrenic nerve between the mediastinal pleura and the fibrous pericardium. Sensory innervation to the pericardium is carried via the phrenic nerves.

Clinical Significance

Pericarditis

Inflammation of the pericardium that may cause chest pain and pericardial friction rub, which can be detected during auscultation.

Pericardial Tamponade

An increase in fluid in the pericardial cavity (e.g., from chronic inflammation) may decrease the efficiency of the heart as it is compressed. Pericardiocentesis is the drainage of excess fluid from the pericardial sac.

Structure of the heart
(Figure 1-6)

The heart is contained within the pericardial sac. It is located within the middle mediastinum, left of the median plane in the thorax. The heart is essentially a cone-shaped muscular pump, the apex of which is directed anteroinferiorly to the left and the base posterolaterally to the right. The base of the heart is the location of the superior vena cava, ascending aorta and pulmonary trunk.

Structure	Description	Significance
Heart surfaces	• Anterior (sternocostal) • Inferior (diaphragmatic) • Right and left pulmonary surfaces	• Anterior—formed mainly by right ventricle • Diaphragmatic—formed mainly by left ventricle (some right ventricle) related to central tendon of diaphragm • Left pulmonary—formed mainly by left ventricle, related to cardiac notch of left lung • Right pulmonary—formed mainly by right atrium
Pectinate muscles	Muscular ridges found on the walls of the atria	• Found in primitive parts of both atria • Presence indicates "rough" part of atrial walls
Trabeculae carneae	Muscular ridges found on the walls of the ventricles	• Found in primitive parts of both ventricles • Serve to increase mechanical advantage during ventricular contraction • Presence indicates "rough" part of ventricular walls

(continued)

Structure of the heart *(continued)*

Structure	Description	Significance
Papillary muscles	Conical muscular projections from the ventricular wall that attach to chordae tendineae	Contract immediately before ventricular contraction to pull chordae tendineae taut to prevent backflow during ventricular contraction (systole)
Chordae tendineae	Attached to margins of atrioventricular valves and papillary muscles	Hold valve cusps taut during ventricular contraction to prevent backflow (regurgitation)
Interatrial septum	Muscular septum separating the atria	Right side—location of fossa ovalis: remnant of foramen ovale, an embryologic shunt for blood from the right atrium to the left atrium
Interventricular septum	Composed of a membranous (superior) part and a muscular (inferior) part	Separates right and left ventricles
Right and left atrioventricular valves	• Right—3 cusps (tricuspid) • Left—2 cusps (bicuspid, mitral)	• Right—permits passage of blood from right atrium to right ventricle and prevents backflow in the reverse direction • Left—permits passage of blood from left atrium to left ventricle and prevents backflow in the reverse direction
Fibrous skeleton	• Collagenous skeleton of heart • Forms fibrous rings that surround heart orifices • Fibrous trigones connect rings	• Provides stability and attachment for valve cusps and muscle fibers • Provides electrical insulation between the atria and ventricles
Right atrium	Forms right border of heart	Receives deoxygenated blood from the superior and inferior vena cavae & coronary sinus
Sinus venarum	Smooth-walled part of right atrium	Formed from incorporation of the embryonic **sinus venosus** during development
Sulcus terminalis	Groove on outside of right atrium	External representation of meeting of primitive atrium and **sinus venarum** derived tissues
Crista terminalis	Ridge on inside of right atrium	Internal representation of meeting of primitive atrium and sinus venarum derived tissues

(continued)

Structure of the heart *(continued)*

Structure	Description	Significance
Right auricle	Small, conical projection from right atrium	Remnant of primitive right atrium
Left atrium	Forms most of base of heart	Receives oxygenated blood from 4 pulmonary veins
Left auricle	Finger-like projection from left atrium	Remnant of primitive left atrium
Right ventricle	Forms inferior border of heart	Receives blood from right atrium
Conus arteriosus (infundibulum)	Smooth-walled superior aspect of right ventricle	Entry to the pulmonary trunk
Supraventricular crest	Muscular ridge on inside of right ventricle	Separates rough part of chamber from smooth-walled part of chamber
Septomarginal trabecula (moderator band)	Muscular ridge that extends from the inferior aspect of the interventricular septum to the base of the anterior-most papillary muscle	Conveys right atrioventricular bundle—part of conduction system, to the anterior papillary muscle
Pulmonary valve	• 3 semilunar cusps • Located at apex of conus arteriosus	Prevents backflow (regurgitation) of blood during ventricular relaxation (diastole)
Pulmonary sinuses	Located between cup-shaped semilunar valve leaflets and dilated pulmonary trunk wall	Prevent valve cusps from sticking to pulmonary trunk wall during ventricular contraction
Left ventricle	Forms apex and left border of heart	Thicker wall (4×) than right ventricle because it pumps against greater pressure
Aortic vestibule	Smooth-walled superior aspect of left ventricle	Entry to ascending aorta
Aortic valve	• 3 semilunar cusps • Located near origin of ascending aorta	Prevent backflow (regurgitation) of blood during ventricular relaxation (diastole)
Aortic sinuses	Located between cup-shaped semilunar valve leaflets and dilated ascending aorta wall	• Prevent valve cusps from sticking to ascending aorta wall during ventricular contraction • Right and left sinus give origin to the right and left coronary arteries respectively

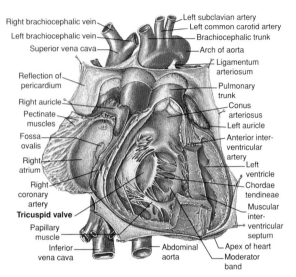

Right brachiocephalic vein
Left brachiocephalic vein
Superior vena cava
Reflection of pericardium
Right auricle
Pectinate muscles
Fossa ovalis
Right atrium
Right coronary artery
Tricuspid valve
Papillary muscle
Inferior vena cava

Left subclavian artery
Left common carotid artery
Brachiocephalic trunk
Arch of aorta
Ligamentum arteriosum
Pulmonary trunk
Conus arteriosus
Left auricle
Anterior interventricular artery
Left ventricle
Chordae tendineae
Muscular interventricular septum
Apex of heart
Moderator band
Abdominal aorta

FIGURE 1-5. Heart. Right interior view. (Asset provided by Anatomical Chart Company.)

Additional Concept

Heart is a "Double Pump"

Right side of the heart: right atrium receives deoxygenated blood from the vena cavae; the right ventricle pumps this blood to the lungs for oxygenation via the pulmonary trunk. Left side of the heart: left atrium receives oxygenated blood from the pulmonary veins; the left ventricle pumps this blood to the body via the aorta.

Walls of the Heart

The walls of all 4 chambers of the heart consist of the same three layers from superficial to deep:

epicardium—layer of mesothelium; also known as visceral layer of serous pericardium

myocardium—middle layer composed of cardiac muscle tissue

endocardium—layer of endothelium that lines heart chambers and valves

Auscultation

Auscultation of the valves: each of the 4 valves of the heart is heard best at specific locations on the thoracic wall:

bicuspid valve—5th intercostal space on the left
tricuspid valve—4th intercostal space to the left of the sternum
pulmonary valve—2nd intercostal space to the left of the sternum
aortic valve—2nd intercostal space to the right of the sternum

Ventricles

Ventricle characteristics—fewer, larger papillary muscles, more numerous trabeculae carneae, fewer, thicker atrioventricular valve cusps and fewer, thicker chordae tendineae are characteristics of the left ventricle owing to its increased workload relative to the right ventricle.

Clinical Significance

Foramen Ovale

Incomplete closure of the **foramen ovale** occurs in 15%–25% of adults, it is typically asymptomatic.

Septal Defects

The membranous part of the **interventricular septum** is the most common site of interventricular septal defects; severe defects may result in hypertension and cardiac failure.

Nerves of the heart

Nerve	Origin	Structures Innervated
Superficial cardiac plexus	• Sympathetic—sympathetic trunks • Parasympathetic—vagus nerves • Located inferior to the aortic arch and anterior to the right pulmonary artery	• Sympathetic—terminate on SA and AV nodes, increases heart rate and force of contraction, produces vasodilation of coronary arteries • Parasympathetic—terminate on SA and AV nodes and coronary arteries, decreases heart rate and force of contraction, causes vasoconstriction of coronary arteries

(continued)

Nerves of the heart (continued)

Nerve	Origin	Structures Innervated
Deep cardiac plexus	• Sympathetic—sympathetic trunks • Parasympathetic—vagus nerves • Located posterior to the aortic arch and anterior to the tracheal bifurcation	
Visceral afferents of cardiac plexuses	Fibers travel with sympathetics and in the vagus nerve	• Fibers traveling with sympathetics convey pain information to T1–T5 spinal cord segments; these fibers are involved in pain referred to the left upper limb during heart attack • Fibers traveling in the vagus nerve innervate baroreceptors and chemoreceptors that monitor pressure and gas concentrations in the blood
Sinuatrial (SA) node	Group of self-excitable cardiac muscle cells located near the junction of the superior vena cava and the right atrium	Pacemaker of the heart, gives an impulse ~70 times per minute
Atrioventricular (AV) node	Located on the right side of the atrial septum near the opening of the coronary sinus	• Receives impulse from wall of atria that was initiated in the SA node • Passes impulse to ventricles via the AV bundle
AV bundle (Bundle of His)	Fiber bundle passing from the AV node to membranous part of interventricular septum, where it terminates by dividing into bundle branches	Only bridge of conduction system between atria and ventricles
Right and left bundle branches	Formed by termination of AV bundle, follow interventricular septum to ventricular walls where they ramify	• Supply cardiac muscle cells of ventricular walls through ramifications (subendocardial branches) • Right bundle branch sends a branch through the septomarginal trabeculae of the right ventricle to the anterior papillary muscle

Additional Concept

Postsynaptic parasympathetic ganglia are located near the SA and AV nodes.

Vessels of the heart

Artery	Origin	Description
Right coronary	Right aortic sinus	Supplies right atrium & ventricle, left ventricle, SA and AV nodes, and interventricular septum
SA nodal branch	Right coronary artery	Supplies SA node
Right marginal branch		Supplies right ventricle and apex of heart
Posterior interventricular		Supplies both ventricles and posterior aspect of interventricular septum
AV nodal branch		Supplies AV node
Left coronary	Left aortic sinus	Supplies left atrium and ventricle, right ventricle, and interventricular septum
Anterior interventricular (left anterior descending	Left coronary artery	Supplies right and left ventricles and interventricular septum
Left circumflex branch		Supplies left atrium and ventricle
Left marginal branch	Left circumflex branch	Supplies left ventricle
Posterior interventricular branch	Left coronary artery	Supplies interventricular septum

Vein	Termination	Description
Coronary sinus	Right atrium	Large vein on posterior aspect of heart in coronary sulcus; accepts most venous blood from the heart before emptying into right atrium
Great cardiac	Coronary sinus	Runs with anterior interventricular artery in anterior interventricular sulcus; becomes coronary sinus on posterior aspect of heart
Middle cardiac		Runs with posterior interventricular artery in posterior interventricular sulcus
Small cardiac		Runs with right marginal branch
Oblique vein of left atrium		Remnant of primordial left superior vena cava
Left posterior ventricular		Drains posterior aspect of left ventricle
Left marginal		Drains left margin of heart
Anterior cardiac	Right atrium	Drains right ventricle
Smallest cardiac	Chambers of heart	Drains walls of all 4 chambers of heart

Additional Concept

Venous Drainage

Venous drainage of the heart is said to be "indirect" because most venous blood enters the coronary sinus before being emptied into the right atrium.

Clinical Significance

Coronary Arteries

Coronary artery disease is a leading cause of death, typically as a result of decreased blood flow to the heart. An area of myocardium that has undergone necrosis (as a result of lack of blood) constitutes a myocardial infarction or heart attack.

LUNGS AND PLEURA

Structure of the pleural cavities
(Figures 1-4, 1-6 and 1-7)

Structure	Description	Significance
Endothoracic fascia	Fibroareolar layer between parietal pleura and thoracic wall	Invests muscular and skeletal elements of thoracic wall and adheres parietal pleura to inner surface of thoracic wall
Costal pleura	Parietal pleura adherent to the inner surface of the ribs and costal cartilages via the endothoracic fascia	Intercostal and phrenic nerves provide sensory innervation; therefore, pain may be referred to the thoracic wall and neck
Mediastinal pleura	Parietal pleura adherent to the outer surface of the mediastinum via the endothoracic fascia	
Diaphragmatic pleura	Parietal pleura adherent to the superior surface of the diaphragm via the endothoracic fascia	
Cervical pleura	• Parietal pleura extending into the root of the neck • Covered by the suprapleural membrane—a regional thickening of the endothoracic fascia	
Pulmonary ligament	Double-layered fold of pleura extending inferiorly from the root of the lung	Area of reflection—visceral pleura from the surface of the lung is continuous with parietal pleura

(continued)

Structure of the pleural cavities *(continued)*

Structure	Description	Significance
Visceral pleura	Covers all surfaces of each lung	• Continuous with parietal pleura at the root of the lung • No or very limited pain afferents
Pleural cavity	Potential space between the visceral and parietal pleura	• Contains capillary layer of serous fluid • Negative pressure here maintains lungs in inflated state
Left and right costodiaphragmatic recesses	Potential space between costal and diaphragmatic pleura	During inspiration the lungs enter the recesses
Left and right costomediastinal recess	Potential spaces between costal and mediastinal pleura	

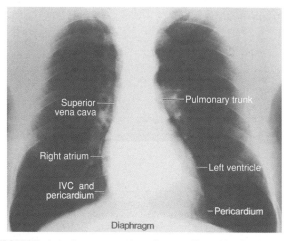

FIGURE 1-6. Anteroposterior chest radiograph. Radiograph shows the various components of the heart and great vessels. (From Dudek RW, Louis TM. *High-Yield Gross Anatomy.* 3rd ed. Baltimore: Lippincott Williams & Wilkins; 2008:85.)

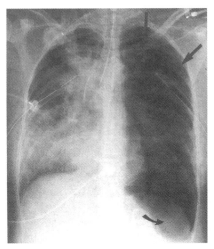

FIGURE 1-7. Pneumothorax. A pneumothorax is air in the plural cavity; this has the effect of collapsing the elastic lung as the negative pressure maintaining it in its expanded state is lost. Posteroanterior radiograph shows a left apical (straight arrows) and subpulmonic (curved arrow) pneumothorax in a 41-year-old woman with respiratory distress syndrome. (From Dudek RW, Louis TM. *High-Yield Gross Anatomy*. 3rd ed. Baltimore: Lippincott Williams & Wilkins; 2008:64.)

Clinical Significance
Cervical Pleura
The **cervical pleura** and apex of the lung are subject to injury from neck wounds because the pleural cavity extends into the root of the neck.

Tracheobronchial tree
(Figure 1-4)

Structure	Description	Significance
Tracheal rings	20 U-shaped hyaline cartilages	• Keep trachea patent • Posteriorly oriented opening of U-shaped cartilage allows for expansion of the esophagus during swallowing

(continued)

Tracheobronchial tree *(continued)*

Structure	Description	Significance
Trachealis	Layer of smooth muscle	Spans posterior deficiency of tracheal rings
Right and left main bronchi	• Extend from tracheal bifurcation to hilum of lungs • Supported by U-shaped hyaline cartilage • Terminate by dividing into lobar bronchi	• Form part of root of the lung • Enter lung at hilum • Right main bronchus is shorter, wider and more vertically oriented than the left • Hyaline cartilage keeps both main bronchi patent
Carina	Keel-like septum projecting superiorly at the bifurcation of the trachea	Visible on radiographs; displacement may indicate thoracic pathology
Lobar (secondary) bronchi (3; right)	• Supported by hyaline cartilage	• Hyaline cartilage keeps lobar bronchi patent
Lobar (secondary) bronchi (2; left)	• Extend from main bronchi until termination as segmental bronchi	• Each lobar bronchus corresponds to a lobe of the lung
Segmental (tertiary) bronchi	• Supported by hyaline cartilage • Formed from terminal branches of lobar bronchi	• Supply bronchopulmonary segments—right lung: 10 segmental bronchi • Left lung: 8–10 segmental bronchi
Bronchopulmonary segments	Pyramidal-shaped with apex directed toward root of lung and base toward outer surface of lung	• Each receives a segmental bronchus and a branch of both pulmonary and bronchial arteries • Intersegmental veins help identify boundaries between segments for resection

Additional Concept

Bronchopulmonary Segments

- Right lung—Superior lobe: Apical, Posterior, Anterior
  Middle lobe: Lateral, Medial
  Inferior lobe: Superior, Anterior basal, Posterior basal, Lateral basal, Medial basal
- Left lung—Superior lobe: Superior division—Apicoposterior, Anterior; Lingular division—Superior, Inferior
  Inferior lobe: superior, Anterior basal, posterior basal, Lateral basal, Medial basal

Mnemonic

Inhale a Bite, Goes Down the Right

Inhaled objects more likely to enter right bronchus, as it is wider, shorter, and more vertical than the left.

Structure of the lungs

The lungs are the elastic organs of respiration. Their function depends upon surface tension in the pleural cavity keeping the parietal and visceral layers of pleura together.

Structure	Description	Significance
Right lung	3 lobes (superior, middle, and inferior) separated by a horizontal and oblique fissure	The right lung is larger than the left
Left lung	2 lobes (superior and inferior) separated by an oblique fissure	The left lung is smaller than the right owing to the position of the heart
Cardiac notch	Indentation of superior lobe of left lung along the anteroinferior border	Result of the heart and pericardial sac bulging to the left
Lingula	Tongue-like process of superior lobe of the left lung inferior to the cardiac notch	
Root of lung	• Formed by pulmonary and bronchial arteries, pulmonary and bronchial veins, lymphatics, nerves, and main bronchi • Enclosed by pleural sleeve	Located on medial aspect of lung, site at which structures enter and leave the lung
Hilum of lung	Located on medial aspect of lungs	Root of lung enters lung here
Horizontal and oblique fissures	• Right lung has 1 horizontal and 1 oblique fissure • Left lung has 1 oblique fissure	Separate lungs into lobes: right lung 3, left lung 2

Nerves of the lungs

Nerve	Origin	Structures Innervated
Anterior pulmonary plexus	• Sympathetic—sympathetic trunks • Parasympathetic—vagus nerves • Located anterior to root of lung	• Sympathetic—inhibit bronchial smooth muscle (bronchodilate) and glands, motor to vessels (vasoconstrict) • Parasympathetic—inhibit vessel musculature (vasodilate), motor to smooth muscle of bronchial tree (bronchoconstrict) and glands (stimulates mucous secretion)
Posterior pulmonary plexus	• Sympathetic—sympathetic trunks • Parasympathetic—vagus nerves • Located posterior to root of lung	
Visceral afferents of pulmonary plexuses	Fibers travel in vagus nerve	Sensory to tissues of the lungs and bronchi—touch, stretch, temperature, and chemical irritants

Additional Concept

Postsynaptic parasympathetic ganglia are found distributed throughout both plexuses.

Vessels of the lungs

Artery	Origin	Description
Right and left pulmonary	Pulmonary trunk	Give rise to lobar arteries; carry deoxygenated blood to the lungs
Lobar	Pulmonary arteries	3 right and 2 left lobar arteries carry deoxygenated blood to each lobe of the lung; accompany secondary bronchi
Right and left bronchial	• Right—posterior intercostal artery • Left—thoracic aorta	Supply oxygenated blood to the tissues of the bronchial tree
Vein	**Termination**	**Description**
Right and left pulmonary	Left atrium	2 pairs of pulmonary veins convey oxygenated blood to the left atrium

(continued)

Vessels of the lungs (continued)

Vein	Termination	Description
Right and left bronchial	• Right—azygos vein • Left—accessory hemiazygos vein	Drain deoxygenated blood from the bronchial tree

Additional Concept

Ligamentum Arteriosum

The **ligamentum arteriosum** is the remnant of the **ductus arteriosus**—an embryologic shunt connecting the arch of the aorta and the left pulmonary artery.

Lymphatics of the lungs

Lymphatic structure	Description	Drainage
Superficial lymphatic plexus	Located immediately deep to visceral pleura	Drains to bronchopulmonary lymph nodes
Deep lymphatic plexus	Located in the submucosa of bronchi and connective tissue around the bronchi	Drains to pulmonary lymph nodes
Pulmonary lymph nodes	Located along the lobar (secondary) bronchi	Drain to bronchopulmonary lymph nodes
Bronchopulmonary (hilar) lymph nodes	Located in the hilum of the lung(s)	Drain to tracheobronchial lymph nodes
Superior and inferior tracheobronchial lymph nodes	Located at the bifurcation of the trachea	Drain to bronchomediastinal trunks (right and left)

Additional Concept

The superficial and deep **lymphatic plexuses** of the lungs communicate freely.

Clinical Significance

Bronchopulmonary nodes are an early site of tumor metastases in bronchogenic carcinoma.

Abdomen

INTRODUCTION

The abdomen is that portion of the trunk inferior to the diaphragm and superior to the pelvis with which it is continuous. The abdomen extends inferiorly to the superior pelvic aperture.

AREAS AND FASCIA OF THE ABDOMEN

Areas of the abdomen

Area	Structure	Significance
Abdominal cavity	Boundaries: • Superior—diaphragm • Inferior—continuous with pelvic cavity at superior pelvic aperture • Anterolateral—muscular abdominal wall • Posterior—vertebral column	Larger, superior part of the abdominopelvic cavity
Regions (9)	Divided into regions by: • 2 horizontal planes—subcostal and transtubercular • 2 vertical-midclavicular planes	• Regions: • Right and left hypochondriac • Right and left inguinal • Right and left lateral • Epigastric • Umbilical • Pubic • Used for description of organ location or location of pathologic processes

(continued)

Areas of the abdomen *(continued)*

Area	Structure	Significance
Quadrants (4)	Divided into quadrants by a horizontal (transumbilical) and a vertical (median) plane	• Quadrants: • Right and left upper • Right and left lower • Used for description of organ location or location of pathologic processes
Inguinal canal	• 4–6 cm long, inferomedially directed passage extending between the deep and superficial inguinal rings • Walls of canal: • Anterior—external oblique aponeurosis • Posterior—transversalis fascia and medially the conjoint tendon • Roof—transversalis fascia and arching fibers of the internal oblique and transversus abdominis • Floor—iliopubic tract, inguinal ligament, and lacunar ligament from lateral to medial	• Transmits the spermatic cord or round ligament of the uterus, ilioinguinal nerve, and the genital branch of the genitofemoral nerve • One result of the oblique nature of canal is that the superficial and deep rings do not overlap; therefore, increases in intra-abdominal pressure force the canal "closed" to prevent herniation
Subinguinal space	Space located deep to the inguinal ligament and iliopubic tract	Serves to connect the abdominopelvic cavity with the lower limb

Additional Concepts

Deep Inguinal Ring

The **deep inguinal** ring, the internal opening of the inguinal canal, is an evagination of transversalis fascia, just superior to the middle of the inguinal ligament and immediately lateral to the inferior epigastric vessels.

Superficial Inguinal Ring

The **superficial inguinal ring** is the slitlike external opening of the inguinal canal in the aponeurosis of the external oblique muscle, just superior to the public tubercle. The medial and lateral margins of the opening are the **medial** and **lateral crura**, which are prevented from spreading apart by **intercrural fibers**.

Structures of the abdominal wall

Feature	Description
Superficial fascia	Inferior to umbilicus, it is composed of 2 layers: • A superficial fatty layer (Camper's fascia) • A deep membranous layer (Scarpa's fascia)
Investing fascia	Covers the muscles (4) forming the muscular wall of the abdomen
Endoabdominal fascia	• Lines inner surface of abdominal wall • Named according to muscle it lines: • **Transversalis fascia** lines the transverse abdominal muscle • Divided into anterior, middle, and posterior layers • Middle and posterior layers enclose the intrinsic muscles of the back—relatively thick, provides attachment for anterolateral abdominal wall muscles • Anterior layer is fascia of quadratus lumborum muscle—thickened superiorly to form **lateral arcuate ligament,** inferiorly attaches to **iliolumbar ligament** • **Lumbar fascia** lines the quadratus lumborum • **Psoas fascia** lines the psoas major muscle • It is thickened superiorly to form the **medial arcuate ligament** • It is continuous with the **thoracolumbar fascia**
Parietal peritoneum	• Lines abdominopelvic cavity • Located deep to the endoabdominal fascia from which it is separated by extraperitoneal fat
Rectus sheath	• Formed by the aponeuroses of the external and internal oblique and transverse abdominal • The sheath contains the rectus abdominis, the superior and inferior epigastric vessels, the pyramidalis, segmental nerves, and lymphatics

(continued)

Structures of the abdominal wall *(continued)*

Feature	Description
Conjoint tendon	• Fused tendons of internal oblique and transverse abdominal at their attachment to the pubis • Forms medial portion of posterior wall of inguinal canal
Inguinal ligament	• Free, fibrous inferior edge of external oblique, extending between the anterior superior iliac spine and pubic tubercle • Laterally provides attachment for transverse abdominal and internal oblique
Iliopubic tract	• Thickened inferior margin of the transversalis fascia • Forms portion of floor and posterior wall of inguinal canal • Located posterior and parallel to the inguinal ligament • Forms the anterior boundary of the **subinguinal space**
Lacunar ligament	• Medial-most internally directed portion of the inguinal ligament • Forms portion of floor of inguinal canal • Attaches to superior pubic ramus
Pectineal ligament	Continuation of lacunar ligament as it runs along the pectin pubis

Additional Concept

Rectus Sheath

Rectus sheath—Above a line midway between the pubic symphysis and umbilicus the anterior layer of the sheath is formed by the external oblique and the anterior portion of the internal oblique, which splits to contribute to the posterior layer of the sheath with the transverse abdominal muscle. Below this line, the sheath is deficient posteriorly, with the aponeurosis of all three muscles forming the anterior layer of the sheath, with only the transversalis fascia separating the rectus abdominis from the parietal peritoneum. The lower edge of the aponeurotic "line" of the posterior sheath is the **arcuate line**.

ABDOMINAL WALL

Muscles of the abdominal wall

Muscle	Proximal Attachment	Distal Attachment	Innervation	Main Actions
Anterolateral Abdominal Wall				
External oblique	Ribs 5–12	Linea alba, pubic crest and tubercle, anterior iliac crest	T5–T12	Compress, protect, and support abdominal contents; flex and rotate trunk
Internal oblique	Thoracolumbar fascia, anterior iliac crest, inguinal ligament	Ribs 10–12, linea alba, pectin pubis (via conjoint tendon)	T6–T12 and L1	Compress, protect, and support abdominal contents
Transverse abdominal	Costal cartilages 7–12, thoracolumbar fascia, iliac crest, inguinal ligament	Linea alba, pubic crest, pectin pubis (via conjoint tendon)		
Rectus abdominis	Pubic symphysis and pubic crest	Xiphoid process, costal cartilages 5–7	T6–T12	Compress, protect, and support abdominal contents; flex trunk (lumbar region)
Pyramidalis	Pubis	Linea alba	T12	Tenses **linea alba**
Spermatic Cord and Scrotum				
Cremaster	Found within cremaster fascia		Genitofemoral	Draws testes closer to body
Dartos	Found within superficial fascia of scrotum		Autonomic	Wrinkles skin of scrotum
Posterior Abdominal Wall				
Psoas minor	T12–L1 vertebrae and intervertebral discs	Pectin pubis	L1	Weak trunk flexor; often absent

(continued)

Muscles of the abdominal wall *(continued)*

Muscle	Proximal Attachment	Distal Attachment	Innervation	Main Actions
Psoas major	T12–L5 vertebrae and intervertebral discs	Lesser trochanter of femur	L2–L4	Together form iliopsoas—the chief flexor of the thigh
Iliacus	Iliac fossa		Femoral	
Quadratus lumborum	12th rib	Iliolumbar ligament and iliac crest	T12–L4	Extends and laterally rotates vertebral column

Skeletal elements (attachments) discussed above are presented with the thorax and pelvis.

Clinical Significance

Guarding Reflex

In addition to the functions mentioned previously, the flat abdominal wall muscles provide protection to abdominal viscera through involuntary contraction when touched or when an underlying structure is inflamed, becoming rigid; this is known as the "guarding" reflex.

Mnemonics

Orientation

Hands-in-your-pockets orientation:

When you put your hands in your pants pockets, your fingers have the orientation of fibers of the external oblique inferomedially.

Internal oblique fibers are at right angles to external oblique fibers.

Psoas Major

Innervation of psoas major: Hitting **L2, L3, and L4** makes the psoas sore.

Vessels of the abdominal wall

Artery	Origin	Description
Musculophrenic	Internal thoracic	Supplies: diaphragm, anterolateral abdominal wall
Superior epigastric		
Inferior epigastric	External iliac	Supplies: rectus abdominis, antero-lateral abdominal wall

(continued)

Vessels of the abdominal wall *(continued)*

Artery	Origin	Description
Superficial epigastric	Femoral	Supplies: region between umbilicus and pubis
Superficial circumflex iliac		Supplies: inguinal region and anterosuperior thigh
Deep circumflex iliac	External iliac	Supplies: iliacus and anterolateral abdominal wall
Subcostal	Thoracic aorta	Supplies: anterolateral abdominal wall
Lumbar (4–5 pairs)	Abdominal aorta	Supplies: back and posterior abdominal wall
Testicular		Supplies: testes and epididymis
Artery of the ductus deferens	Inferior vesical artery	Supplies: ductus deferens
Cremasteric	Inferior epigastric artery	Supplies: cremaster muscle and fascia

Vein	Termination	Description
Pampiniform plexus	Plexus converges to form the testicular veins	Drains the spermatic cord and testes

Additional Concept

Abdominal Aorta

The abdominal aorta is the continuation of the thoracic aorta after it passes through the aortic hiatus of the diaphragm. The abdominal aorta terminates by dividing into common iliac arteries at L4 vertebral level. The abdominal aorta gives:

- paired visceral branches: suprarenal, renal, and gonadal
- unpaired visceral branches: celiac trunk, superior mesenteric and inferior mesenteric arteries
- paired parietal: inferior phrenic and lumbar
- unpaired parietal: median sacral artery.

Venous Drainage

Veins generally parallel arteries and drain into the inferior vena cava, with the notable exception of the portal system, which drains to the liver.

Nerves of the abdominal wall

Nerve	Origin	Structures Innervated
Thoracoabdominals	T7–T11	Anterolateral abdominal wall superior to iliac crest
Subcostal	T12	

(continued)

Nerves of the abdominal wall *(continued)*

Nerve	Origin	Structures Innervated
Lumbar Plexus		
Iliohypogastric	L1	Anterolateral abdominal wall of inguinal and hypogastric regions
Ilioinguinal		Scrotum/labia majorum, mons pubis, medial thigh, and lower-most aspect of anterolateral abdominal wall
Genitofemoral	L1, L2	Divides into genital and femoral branches; genital branch supplies cremaster and cutaneous innervation to anterior aspect of scrotum; femoral branch is sensory to anteromedial aspect of thigh
Lateral cutaneous nerve of the thigh	L2, L3	Supplies sensory innervation to anterolateral aspect of thigh
Obturator	L2–L4	Supplies adductor compartment of thigh
Femoral		Supplies hip flexors and knee extensors
Lumbosacral trunk	L4, L5	Participates in formation of sacral plexus (L4–S4)

Mnemonic

Lumbar Plexus

Lumbar plexus nerve roots: 2 from 1, 2 from 2, 2 from 3:

2 nerves from 1 root: ilioinguinal (L1), iliohypogastric (L1).
2 nerves from 2 roots: genitofemoral (L1–L2), lateral cutaneous nerve of the thigh (L2–L3). 2 nerves from 3 roots: obturator (L2–L4), femoral (L2–L4).

Structure of the scrotum

Feature	Description	Significance
Wall	Double layered: skin and superficial fascia (dartos): contains smooth muscle fibers—dartos muscle	• Outpouching of lower anterior abdominal wall • **Dartos muscle** receives autonomic innervation and functions to wrinkle the skin
Arterial Supply		
Posterior scrotal branches	Origin: perineal artery	Supplies posterior aspect
Anterior scrotal branches	Origin: external pudendal artery	Supplies anterior aspect
Cremaster artery	Origin: inferior epigastric artery	Supplies the superior aspect

(continued)

Structure of the scrotum *(continued)*

Feature	Description	Significance
Nerve Supply		
Genital branch of genitofemoral nerve	Origin: genitofemoral nerve (L1–L2)	Supplies anterolateral surface
Anterior scrotal nerves	Origin: ilioinguinal nerve (L1)	Supplies anterior surface
Posterior scrotal nerves	Origin: perineal branches of pudendal nerve (S1–S4)	Supplies posterior surface
Perineal branches of posterior femoral cutaneous	Origin: posterior femoral cutaneous nerve (S2–S3)	Supplies inferior surface

The testes and epididymis are presented with the reproductive organs in the pelvis and perineum chapter.

Clinical Significance

Sensory Innervation of the Scrotum

As the anterior aspect of the scrotum is supplied by branches of the ilioinguinal nerve and the posterior aspect by the branches of the perineal and posterior femoral cutaneous nerves, care must be taken to properly anesthetize the scrotum for surgical procedures.

Structure of the spermatic cord

The spermatic cord runs through the inguinal canal into the scrotum. The cord contains structures coursing between the scrotum and the abdominopelvic cavity.

Structure	Description	Significance
Fascial coverings of spermatic cord	• Internal—internal spermatic fascia • Middle—cremaster fascia • External—external spermatic fascia	• Internal spermatic—derived from transversalis fascia • **Cremaster**—derived from internal oblique • External spermatic—derived from external oblique

(continued)

Structure of the spermatic cord *(continued)*

Structure	Description	Significance
Components		
Ductus deferens	Tube composed of smooth muscle	Conveys sperm from the epididymis to the ejaculatory duct
Testicular artery	Arises from abdominal aorta	Supplies testes and epididymis
Artery of the ductus deferens	Arises from inferior vesical artery	Supplies ductus deferens
Cremasteric artery	Arises from inferior epigastric artery	Supplies cremaster muscle and fascia
Pampiniform plexus of veins	Venous plexus that drains the testes and spermatic cord	Converges to form the testicular veins
Autonomics	Sympathetic and parasympathetic nerve network	• Innervates dartos and vessels of region • Responsible for peristaltic contractions during emission
Genital branch of genitofemoral	Origin: L1–L2; divides into genital and femoral branches	Supplies cremaster muscle

Clinical Significance

Temperature Regulation

The **cremaster muscle** (skeletal muscle), found with the cremaster fascia, draws the testes toward the body in cold temperatures as part of the cremasteric reflex. The **dartos muscle** (smooth muscle) causes wrinkling of the scrotum to draw the testes nearer the body and reduce the surface area of the scrotum in cold temperatures.

PERITONEAL CAVITY

Structure of the peritoneal cavity
(Figure 2-1)

The peritoneal cavity is a potential, fluid-filled space between adjacent layers of peritoneum in the abdomen. It is divided into a lesser and a greater sac that correspond to their embryologic origins as the right and left halves of the intraembryonic cavity.

Structure of the peritoneal cavity *(continued)*

Feature	Description	Significance
Lesser sac (omental bursa)	Bounded by: • Anterior—liver, stomach and lesser omentum • Posterior—diaphragm • Right—liver • Left—gastrosplenic and gastrorenal ligaments	• Smaller portion of the peritoneal cavity • Formed by embryologic rotation of the gut
Superior recess of lesser sac	Limited by diaphragm and posterior leaf of coronary ligament of the liver	Superior extent of the lesser sac
Inferior recess of lesser sac	Limited by fusion of anterior and posterior leafs of greater omentum	Inferior extent of the lesser sac
Greater sac	All of the peritoneal cavity that is not the lesser sac	• Larger portion of the peritoneal cavity • Formed by embryologic rotation of the gut
Omental foramen	Located posterior to the portal triad and anterior to the inferior vena cava	Connection between the lesser and greater sac
Paracolic gutters	Depressions running parallel with the ascending and descending colon along the posterior abdominal wall	• Function as channels that convey peritoneal fluid • Communication between supra- and infracolic compartments
Supracolic compartment	Formed by the mesentery of the transverse colon—the transverse mesocolon	Part of the peritoneal cavity superior to the transverse mesocolon
Infracolic compartment		Part of the peritoneal cavity inferior to the transverse mesocolon
Subphrenic spaces	Superior extensions of the peritoneal cavity between the diaphragm and liver	Separated into right and left by the falciform ligament
Hepatorenal recess	Extension of peritoneal cavity inferior to the liver and anterior to the kidney and suprarenal gland	• Communicates anteriorly with the right subphrenic space • Communicates with omental bursa (lesser sac)—fluid may drain into recess from here when supine

(continued)

Feature	Description	Significance
Peritoneal Fossae		
Supravesical fossae	Between the median and medial umbilical folds	Potential site for a hernia
Medial inguinal fossae (related to inguinal triangles)	Between the medial and lateral umbilical folds	Potential site for a **direct inguinal hernia**
Lateral inguinal fossae	Lateral to the lateral umbilical folds	Deep inguinal rings found within fossae, potential site for **indirect inguinal hernia**

Peritoneal pouches are presented with the pelvis.

Clinical Significance

Peritoneal Puncture

Occasionally it is necessary to puncture the peritoneum to remove excess fluid (ascites) that accumulates during inflammation, to conduct peritoneal dialysis or administer anesthetic agents through intraperitoneal injection.

Peritoneum
(Figure 2-1)

Structure	Description	Significance
Parietal peritoneum	Serous membrane lining the peritoneal cavity	Lines internal surface of abdominal wall
Visceral peritoneum		Lines external surfaces of abdominal organs
Mesentery	• Double layer of peritoneum connecting intraperitoneal organs to the abdominal wall • Conveys neurovascular elements and lymphatics • Allows movement of the organ to which it is attached	• The "mesentery" refers specifically to the mesentery of the small intestine • Other mesenteries are named specifically for the organs to which they are associated (e.g., transverse mesocolon or mesoappendix)
Peritoneal Folds		
Median umbilical fold	Fold of parietal peritoneum extending from the apex of the bladder to the umbilicus	Covers the **median umbilical ligament**—the remnant of the urachus
Medial umbilical folds (2)	Fold of parietal peritoneum found lateral to the median umbilical fold	Covers the **medial umbilical ligaments**—the obliterated part of the umbilical arteries

(continued)

Peritoneum *(continued)*

Structure	Description	Significance
Lateral umbilical folds (2)	Fold of parietal peritoneum found lateral to the medial umbilical folds	Covers the **inferior epigastric vessels**
Omenta		
Greater	Double layer of peritoneum connecting greater curvature of stomach and proximal duodenum to adjacent organs	3 parts: 1. **Gastrophrenic ligament**—connects stomach to diaphragm 2. **Gastrosplenic ligament**—connects stomach to spleen 3. **Gastrocolic ligament**—connects stomach to transverse colon, largest part, anterior and posterior layers are fused to form a 4-layered structure
Lesser	• Double layer of peritoneum connecting lesser curvature of the stomach and proximal duodenum to adjacent organs • Forms anterior wall of lesser sac	2 parts: 1. **Hepatogastric ligament**—connects stomach to liver 2. **Hepatoduodenal ligament**—connects duodenum to liver, contains **portal triad:** portal vein, hepatic artery and bile duct
Associated with the Liver		
Falciform ligament	• Double layer of peritoneum extending from umbilicus to liver on anterior abdominal wall • Continuous superiorly as left and right coronary ligament	• Embryologic remnant of the ventral mesentery • Contains round ligament of the liver in its inferior, crescentic border
Coronary ligaments (anterior and posterior)	• Anterior formed by separation of leafs of falciform ligament • Posterior is formed of peritoneal reflexion from diaphragm to liver	Bound the **bare area of the liver**
Triangular ligaments (right and left)	Formed of anterior and posterior coronary ligaments	Formed of a peritoneal reflexion between anterior and posterior leafs of coronary ligaments
Round ligament of liver	Connective tissue cord in inferior border of falciform ligament	Embryologic remnant of the umbilical vein

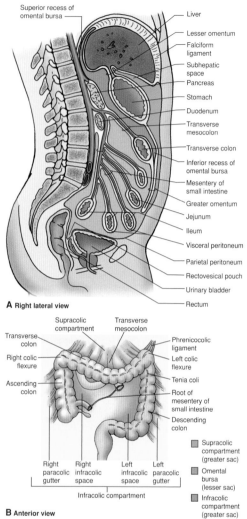

A Right lateral view

B Anterior view

FIGURE 2-1. Subdivisions of peritoneal cavity. **A:** This median section of the abdominopelvic cavity shows the subdivisions of the peritoneal cavity. **B:** The supracolic and infracolic compartments of the greater sac are shown after removal of the greater omentum. The infracolic spaces and paracolic gutters determine the flow of ascitic fluid when inclined or upright. (From Moore KL, Dalley AF. *Clinically Oriented Anatomy.* 5th ed. Baltimore: Lippincott Williams & Wilkins; 2006:239.)

Additional Concepts

Peritoneal Relations

Organs that are suspended by a mesentery are said to be **intraperitoneal**. Organs that lack a mesentery and are only partially covered with peritoneum are said to be **extraperitoneal** (retroperitoneal or subperitoneal provides more indication of their location).

Median Umbilical Ligament

The **median umbilical ligament** is formed by the **urachus**, the obliterated portion of the allantois, connecting the apex of the bladder with the umbilicus.

Medial Umbilical Ligaments

The **medial umbilical ligaments** are formed by the obliterated portions of the **umbilical arteries** distal to the superior vesical arteries.

Clinical Significance

Herniae

A **direct inguinal hernia** (acquired) exits the abdomen via the **medial inguinal fossa** or **inguinal triangle**, which is bounded medially by the semilunar line (lateral border of rectus abdominis), laterally by the lateral umbilical folds and inferiorly by the inguinal ligament.

An **indirect inguinal hernia** (congenital) exits the abdomen via the **deep inguinal ring** and passes through the **inguinal canal** into the scrotum.

Adhesions

Adhesions may develop in the peritoneal cavity as a result of inflammation of the peritoneum (peritonitis) or previous surgery, which may need to be removed if they compromise the function of the viscera.

Mnemonic

Structures forming folds: **IOU**:
From lateral to medial:

lateral umbilical ligament: **I**nferior epigastric vessels
medial umbilical ligament: **O**bliterated umbilical artery
median umbilical ligament: **U**rachus

ESOPHAGUS

Structure of the esophagus

The esophagus is a muscular tube extending from the cricoid cartilage to the gastroesophageal junction; it enters the abdomen through the esophageal hiatus of the diaphragm. The nature of the musculature of the esophagus changes throughout its course:

- upper third—skeletal muscle
- middle third—mixture of smooth and skeletal muscle
- lower third—smooth muscle

Feature	Description	Significance
Sphincters	2 sphincters: 1. Upper esophageal sphincter—skeletal muscle 2. Lower esophageal sphincter—smooth muscle and skeletal muscle of diaphragm	• Upper sphincter composed mainly of **cricopharyngeus** • Lower sphincter—smooth muscle and muscular diaphragmatic esophageal hiatus prevent gastroesophageal reflux
Innervation	• Skeletal muscle part—recurrent branches of the vagus nerve • Smooth muscle part—esophageal plexus	**Esophageal plexus**—parasympathetic fibers from the vagus nerves and sympathetic fibers from sympathetic chain and greater splanchnic nerve
Arterial supply	Inferior thyroid, esophageal, bronchial, left gastric and left inferior phrenic arteries	Arterial supply is generally via whatever arteries lie near this long longitudinally oriented structure
Venous drainage	Esophageal veins empty into the inferior thyroid, azygos, hemiazygos and gastric veins	Important contributor to the portal-caval anastomosis

Clinical Significance

Esophageal Varices

Esophageal varices are dilated esophageal veins that may rupture in cases of portal hypertension.

Pyrosis

Pyrosis (heartburn) is usually the result of regurgitation of stomach contents into the lower esophagus.

STOMACH

Structure of the stomach
(Figure 2-3)

The stomach is the muscular organ of digestion; it produces chyme through enzymatic digestion.

Feature	Description	Significance
Parts		
Cardia	Part surrounding cardial orifice	**Cardial orifice**—funnel-shaped opening of stomach that receives the esophagus
Fundus	Part superior to cardial orifice	Typically dilated and gas-filled
Body	Part between fundus and pyloric antrum	Major part of the stomach
Pylorus	• Distal-most part of the stomach • Possesses smooth muscle sphincter—**pyloric sphincter**, which guards the **pyloric orifice** that opens into the duodenum • Funnel-shaped • Divided into the **pyloric antrum** (wide) and **pyloric canal** (narrow)	Pyloric sphincter controls release of gastric contents into the duodenum and prevents reflux from duodenum into stomach
Curvatures		
Greater	Directed inferior and to the left	Longer, convex curvature
Lesser	Directed superior and to the right	• Shorter, concave curvature • Bears the **angular incisure**—outer representation of the junction of the body and pyloric part
Interior		
Rugae (gastric folds)	Longitudinal folds of gastric mucosa	Function to increase surface area and allow for distension

Clinical Significance

Pylorospasm

Pylorospasm is the failure of the pyloric sphincter to relax, which prevents food from passing from the stomach to the duodenum, often occurs in infants and may result in vomiting.

Vessels of the stomach
(Figure 2-4)

Artery	Origin	Description
Celiac trunk	Abdominal aorta	• Supplies embryologic foregut • Gives rise to: splenic, hepatic and left gastric arteries
Splenic	Celiac trunk	• Supplies the spleen • Gives rise to left gastro-omental and short gastric arteries to the stomach
Hepatic		• Supplies the liver • Gives rise to gastroduodenal and right gastric arteries to the stomach
Gastroduodenal	Hepatic	• Supplies the stomach, duodenum and liver • Gives rise to right gastro-omental to the stomach
Right gastric		Supplies lesser curvature of the stomach
Left gastric	Celiac trunk	
Right gastro-omental	Gastroduodenal	Supplies greater curvature of the stomach
Left gastro-omental	Splenic	Supply body of stomach
Short gastric		
Vein	**Termination**	**Description**
Left gastric	Portal	Drain lesser curvature of stomach
Right gastric		
Left gastro-omental	Splenic	Drain greater curvature of stomach
Right gastro-omental	Superior mesenteric	
Short	Splenic	Drain body of stomach

Nerves of the stomach

Nerve	Origin	Structures Innervated
Parasympathetic	Vagus nerves	Anterior and posterior vagal trunks enter abdomen through the esophageal hiatus
Sympathetic	Presynaptics originate from the intermedio-lateral cell column of the spinal cord and travel in the sympathetic trunks and splanchnic nerves to reach abdominal plexuses	• Presynaptic sympathetics are conveyed to the celiac plexus/ganglia • Postsynaptic fibers travel on branches of the celiac trunk to the stomach • Reduces motility, activates sphincters, vasoconstricts and decreases glandular activity
Visceral afferent	Cell bodies located in spinal ganglia	Stomach sensitive to stretching and distension

SMALL INTESTINE

Structure of the small intestine
(Figures 2-3 and 2-5)

The small intestine extends from the pylorus to the cecum. It is the primary site of digestion and absorption in the body. The small intestine is divided into three parts:

1. duodenum
2. jejunum
3. ileum

Structure	Description	Significance
Duodenum	• 1st part of small intestine • Divided into 4 parts: 1. Superior 2. Descending 3. Horizontal 4. Ascending • Superior part is intraperitoneal, the remaining parts are retroperitoneal	• Descending part receives the bile and main pancreatic ducts via hepatopancreatic ampulla • Ascending part continuous with jejunum at duodenojejunal junction • 1st part referred to as duodenal cap/bulb

(continued)

Structure of the small intestine *(continued)*

Structure	Description	Significance
Duodenojejunal junction	Junction of duodenum and jejunum, evidenced by the duodenojejunal flexure	The sharp angle of the duodenojejunal flexure is supported by the suspensory muscle of the duodenum (ligament of Treitz)—a slip of fibromuscular tissue that supports the flexure
Jejunum	• 2nd part of the small intestine • Intraperitoneal, connected to the posterior abdominal wall by the mesentery	Constitutes ~2/5 of the small intestine distal to the duodenum
Ileum	• 3rd part of the small intestine • Intraperitoneal, connected to the posterior abdominal wall by the mesentery	Constitutes the distal part of the small intestine, extending from the jejunum to the ileocecal junction
Ileocecal junction	Junction of the ileum and the cecum	Invagination of the ileum into the cecum forms folds superior and inferior to the ileal orifice, forming the ileocecal valve

Additional Concept

Distinguishing Characteristics between the Jejunum and Ileum

The jejunum has greater vascularity, longer vasa recta, fewer and larger arterial arcades, less fat in the mesentery, more prominent plicae circulares, and fewer lymphatic elements than the ileum.

Vessels of the small intestine
(Figure 2-3)

The celiac trunk and gastroduodenal arteries are presented with the vessels of the stomach.

Artery	Origin	Description
Superior pancreaticoduodenal	Gastroduodenal	Supplies proximal part of duodenum

(continued)

Vessels of the small intestine *(continued)*

Artery	Origin	Description
Superior mesenteric	Abdominal aorta	• Supplies alimentary canal to left colic flexure • Supplies embryologic midgut
Inferior pancreaticoduodenal	Superior mesenteric	Supplies distal part of duodenum
Arterial arcades		Gives rise to vasa recta that supply the jejunum and ileum

Additional Concept

Venous Drainage

Venous drainage parallels arterial supply and terminates in the portal vein.

Embryologic Arterial Supply

The descending part of the duodenum marks the transition between the embryologic foregut and midgut, the location is marked by anastomosis of branches of the celiac trunk (artery of the foregut) with branches of the superior mesenteric artery (artery of the midgut).

Nerves of the small intestine

Nerve	Origin	Structures Innervated
Parasympathetic	Vagal—primarily the posterior vagal trunk	• Presynaptic parasympathetic fibers synapse in the myenteric and submucosal plexuses in the wall of the small intestine • Increases motility and glandular secretion and inhibits sphincters
Sympathetic	Presynaptics originate from the intermediolateral cell column of the spinal cord and travel in the sympathetic trunks and splanchnic nerves to reach abdominal plexuses	• Presynaptic sympathetics are conveyed to the celiac and superior mesenteric plexuses/ganglia • Postsynaptic fibers travel on branches of the superior mesenteric artery to the small intestine • Reduces motility, activates sphincters, vasoconstricts and decreases glandular activity

(continued)

Nerves of the small intestine *(continued)*

Nerve	Origin	Structures Innervated
Visceral afferent	Cell bodies located in spinal ganglia	Small intestine sensitive to stretching, distension, and pain

LARGE INTESTINE

Structure of the large intestine
(Figure 2-2)

The large intestine extends from the ileocecal junction to the anus. It is divided into four parts:

1. cecum
2. colon
3. rectum
4. anal canal

The large intestine is the part of the digestive tract distal to the small intestine; it is primarily responsible for water and electrolyte resorption.

Structure	Description	Significance
Parts		
Cecum	• 1st part of large intestine • Continuous with ascending colon • Ileum joins it at ileocecal junction	Mostly covered by visceral peritoneum, although has no mesentery
Appendix	• Diverticulum extending from cecum • Possesses a mesentery— mesoappendix	Variable location, but usually is posterior to the cecum
Colon	• 2nd part of large intestine • Divided into 4 parts: 1. Ascending colon extends from cecum to right colic flexure 2. Transverse colon extends from right colic flexure to left colic flexure 3. Descending colon extends from left colic flexure to sigmoid colon 4. Sigmoid colon follows an S-shaped course to the rectum	• The ascending and descending colon are retro-peritoneal, although they are only loosely fixed to the posterior abdominal wall by a loose connective tissue fascia—**fusion fascia** and, therefore, easily mobilized during surgery • On the lateral aspects, are the paracolic gutters • The transverse and sigmoid colon each have mesenteries— the transverse and sigmoid mesocolons

(continued)

Structure of the large intestine *(continued)*

Structure	Description	Significance
Rectum	• 3rd part of large intestine • Extends from the sigmoid colon at S3 to the anal canal • Possesses 3 lateral flexures that correspond to 3 transverse rectal folds, which correspond to thickenings of the muscular wall	• Dilated terminal portion—the ampulla, retains feces until defecation • The proximal third of the rectum is covered by peritoneum on the anterior and lateral aspect, the middle third only has peritoneum on the anterior surface, whereas the inferior 3rd is subperitoneal
Anal canal	• 4th part of large intestine • Begins at the anorectal flexure at the level of the pelvic diaphragm and extends to the anus • Internally possesses anal columns—longitudinal ridges joined at their base by anal valves, anal glands open into the anal sinuses (recesses formed by anal valves)	• The **anorectal flexure** is the primary structure that maintains fecal continence, it is a sharp bend maintained by tonic contraction of **puborectalis;** its relaxation is necessary if defecation is to occur • Feces compressing the anal sinuses causes exudation of mucus that lubricates the anal canal
Features		
Teniae coli	3 longitudinally oriented bands of smooth muscle of the large intestine	The longitudinal layer of smooth muscle surrounding the digestive tract is reduced to 3 bands over the large intestine
Haustra	Sacculations of the large intestine	Slow the passage of feces through the large intestine
Omental appendices	Small, fatty projections hanging from the wall of the large intestine	Allow for reduced friction with nearby structures during movement of the large intestine as feces passes through

Additional Concept

Differences between the Small and Large Intestine

The large intestine has a larger diameter than the small intestine and possesses teniae coli, haustra and omental appendices, all of which are unique to the large intestine.

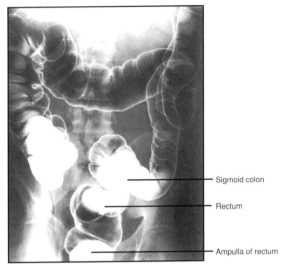

Sigmoid colon

Rectum

Ampulla of rectum

FIGURE 2-2. Anteroposterior barium radiograph showing parts of the large intestine; note the haustra and flexures of the colon. (From Dudek RW, Louis TM. *High-Yield Gross Anatomy.* 3rd ed. Baltimore: Lippincott Williams & Wilkins; 2008:138.)

Clinical Significance

McBurney's Point

Usual location of proximal (open end) of the appendix, located one third of the way along an oblique line connecting the anterior superior iliac spine to the umbilicus.

Sphincters of Anal Canal

The anal canal is surrounded by two sphincters, both of which are involved in the maintenance of fecal continence, the internal (involuntary) and external (voluntary, divided into deep, superficial, and subcutaneous parts) anal sphincters.

Pectinate Line

The inferior border of the anal valves forms the **pectinate line.** Above the pectinate line, the anal canal is derived from the embryologic hindgut (visceral—autonomic innervation, inferior mesenteric arterial supply, venous drainage to portal system, and lymphatics to internal iliac nodes), below the line it is derived from the proctodeum (somatic—somatic innervation, internal iliac arterial supply, venous drainage to caval system, and lymphatics to inguinal nodes).

Teniae Coli

Proximally, the teniae coli converge at the base of the appendix and thereby aid in location of the appendix during surgery.

Vessels of the large intestine

Artery	Origin	Description
Superior mesenteric	Abdominal aorta	• Supplies alimentary canal to left colic flexure • Supplies embryologic midgut
Ileocolic	Superior mesenteric	• Supplies cecum • Gives rise to appendicular artery
Appendicular	Ileocolic	Supplies appendix
Right colic	Superior mesenteric	Supplies ascending colon
Middle colic		Supplies transverse colon
Inferior mesenteric	Abdominal aorta	• Supplies alimentary canal to the anal canal • Supplies embryologic hindgut
Left colic	Inferior mesenteric	Supplies descending colon
Sigmoid		Supplies sigmoid colon
Marginal	Ileocolic, right colic, middle colic, left colic, and sigmoids	Anastomotic loop forming collateral circulation along the large intestine
Superior rectal	Inferior mesenteric	Superior aspect of rectum
Middle rectal	Inferior vesical (male) or uterine (female)	Mid and inferior aspect of rectum
Inferior rectal	Internal pudendal	Anal canal

Additional Concept

Venous Drainage

Venous drainage parallels arterial supply and terminates in the portal vein until the level of the junction of the superior and middle aspects of the rectum; inferior to this point, venous drainage is to the caval system.

Nerves of the large intestine

Nerve	Origin	Structures Innervated
Large Intestine Proximal to Pectinate Line of Anal Canal		
Parasympathetic	• Vagal—to the mid-transverse colon • S2–S4 via pelvic splanchnic nerves	• Presynaptic parasympathetic fibers synapse in the in the wall of the large intestine • Increases motility and glandular secretion and inhibits sphincters
Sympathetic	Presynaptics originate from the intermediolateral cell column of the spinal cord and travel in the sympathetic trunks and splanchnic nerves to reach abdominal plexuses	• Postsynaptic fibers travel on branches of superior and inferior mesenteric arteries to the large intestine • Reduces motility, activates sphincters, vasoconstricts and decreases glandular activity
Visceral afferent	Cell bodies located in spinal ganglia	• Large intestine sensitive to pain, stretching and distension • Afferents involved in reflexes travel with the vagus nerve
Large Intestine Distal to Pectinate Line of Anal Canal		
Inferior rectal	Pudendal	• Somatic innervation • Anal canal inferior to pectinate line

Structure of the liver
(Figures 2-3 and 2-5)

The liver is the largest internal organ and the largest gland in the body. It is surrounded by a connective tissue capsule—**Glisson's capsule**. The liver is divided into anatomic lobes:

- right
- left
- caudate
- quadrate

Functional units of the liver are called **hepatic lobules**— plates of hepatocytes surrounded by sinusoids, which are organized around **portal triads**. The liver receives all substances absorbed by the digestive tract (except lipids), stores glycogen, and secretes bile.

Structure of the liver (continued)

Structure	Description	Significance
Anatomic Lobes		
Right	Located to the right of the right sagittal fissure	Demarcated by the left and right sagittal fissures and the porta hepatis
Left	Located to the left of the left sagittal fissure	
Caudate	Between the left and right sagittal fissures, posterior to the porta hepatis	
Quadrate	Between the left and right sagittal fissures, anterior to the porta hepatis	
Features		
Porta hepatis	Fissure on inferior aspect of liver where structures enter and leave that are enclosed in the hepatoduodenal ligament	• Structures passing through the porta hepatis include: 1. Common bile duct 2. Portal vein 3. Hepatic artery 4. Lymphatics • The first 3 structures compose the **portal triad**
Bare area	• Area on posterior aspect of liver that lacks peritoneum • Bounded by the coronary ligaments	Provides potential route of infection between the abdominal and thoracic cavities
Left sagittal fissure	• Fissure on inferior aspect of liver • Separates the left lobe from the quadrate and caudate lobes	Contains: • **Ligamentum venosum**—remnant of **ductus venosus,** an embryologic shunt for blood • Round ligament—remnant of umbilical vein
Right sagittal fissure	• Fissure on inferior aspect of liver • Separates quadrate and caudate lobes from right lobe of liver	Contains: • Inferior vena cava in the groove for the inferior vena cava • Gall bladder in the fossa of the gall bladder
Right and left hepatic ducts	Drain bile from the right and left lobes	• Right and left bile ducts join inferior to the liver to form the common hepatic duct • Release of bile into the hepatopancreatic ampulla is controlled by the **sphincter of the bile duct**

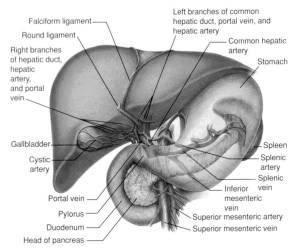

FIGURE 2-3. Liver. Anterior view. (Asset provided by Anatomical Chart Company.)

The remainder of the biliary tree is presented with the gall bladder and pancreas.

Additional Concept

Functional Divisions of the Liver

The liver can also be divided functionally into right and left functional lobes, based on the branching pattern of the right and left hepatic arteries.

Clinical Significance

Cirrhosis

Cirrhosis of the liver is characterized by the replacement of healthy liver cells with fat and fibrous tissue; it is most commonly seen in alcoholics and is a common cause of portal hypertension.

LIVER

Vessels of the liver
(Figures 2-3 and 2-4)

Artery	Origin	Description
Celiac trunk	Abdominal aorta	• Gives rise to splenic, hepatic, and left gastric arteries • Supplies embryologic foregut
Hepatic	Celiac trunk	• Supplies the liver • Gives rise to right and left hepatic arteries
Right and left hepatic	Hepatic	Supply right and left lobes of liver

Vein	Termination	Description
Right, middle and left hepatic	Inferior vena cava	• Drain into inferior vena cava immediately inferior to the diaphragm • Help to hold liver in place
Portal	Sinusoids of liver	• Formed by the junction of the splenic and superior mesenteric veins, which typically receive the inferior mesenteric vein • Conveys all venous blood and absorbed nutrients from the digestive tract from the inferior aspect of the esophagus to the anal canal

Clinical Significance

Portal Hypertension

Portal hypertension is indicated by a rise in pressure in the portal vein and is often caused by cirrhosis, characterized by scarring and fibrosis of the liver. This causes blood to flow into the systemic (caval) system at sites of portal-systemic anastomosis, producing varicose veins.

Nerves of the liver

Nerve	Origin	Structures Innervated
Parasympathetic	Vagus nerves	Anterior and posterior vagal trunks enter abdomen through the esophageal hiatus
Sympathetic	Presynaptics originate in the intermedio-lateral cell column of the spinal cord and travel in the sympathetic trunks and splanchnic nerves to reach abdominal plexuses	• Presynaptic sympathetics are conveyed to the celiac and hepatic plexus • Postsynaptic fibers travel on branches of the hepatic artery to the liver

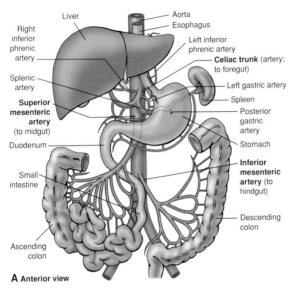

Liver — Aorta — Esophagus

Right inferior phrenic artery

Left inferior phrenic artery

Celiac trunk (artery; to foregut)

Splenic artery — Left gastric artery

Spleen

Superior mesenteric artery (to midgut)

Posterior gastric artery

Duodenum — Stomach

Small intestine — **Inferior mesenteric artery** (to hindgut)

Descending colon

Ascending colon

A Anterior view

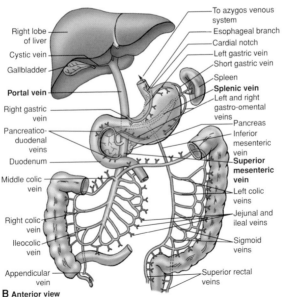

To azygos venous system

Esophageal branch

Cardial notch

Right lobe of liver

Left gastric vein

Cystic vein — Short gastric vein

Gallbladder — Spleen

Splenic vein

Portal vein — Left and right gastro-omental veins

Right gastric vein — Pancreas

Pancreatico-duodenal veins

Inferior mesenteric vein

Duodenum — **Superior mesenteric vein**

Middle colic vein — Left colic veins

Right colic vein — Jejunal and ileal veins

Ileocolic vein — Sigmoid veins

Appendicular vein — Superior rectal veins

B Anterior view

GALL BLADDER

Structure of the gall bladder
(Figures 2-3 and 2-5)

The gall bladder is a pear-shaped organ located in the anterior aspect of the right sagittal fissure of the liver in the gall bladder fossa. It stores and concentrates bile.

Structure	Description	Significance
Fundus	Expanded anterior-most end	Located near the 9th costal cartilage in the midclavicular line
Body	Located between the fundus and neck	In contact with inferior surface of liver
Neck	Narrow posterior-most part; directed toward porta hepatis	Makes S-shaped bend to join cystic duct

Additional Concept

Extrahepatic Duct System

The **cystic duct** of the gall bladder joins the **common hepatic duct**—formed by the junction of the **right** and **left hepatic ducts**—to form the **common bile duct.** The cystic duct drains bile from the gall bladder and the mucosa of the cystic duct is folded in a spiral fashion to form the **spiral valve**, which functions to keep the duct open. The hepatic ducts function to drain bile from the liver. The common bile duct ends at the **hepatopancreatic ampulla**, where it joins the **main pancreatic duct**; release of contents into the duodenum is controlled by the **sphincter of the hepatopancreatic ampulla**—sympathetic innervation causes the sphincter to contract. The remainder of the biliary tree is presented with the liver and pancreas.

FIGURE 2-4. Arterial supply and venous drainage of GI tract. **A:** The arterial supple is demonstrated. **B:** The venous drainage is shown. The portal vein drains poorly oxygenated, nutrient-rich blood from the gastrointestinal tract, spleen, pancreas, and gall-bladder to the liver. The *black arrow* indicates the communication of the esophageal vein with the azygos (systemic) venous system. (From Moore KL, Dalley AF. *Clinically Oriented Anatomy.* 5th ed. Baltimore: Lippincott Williams & Wilkins; 2006:245.)

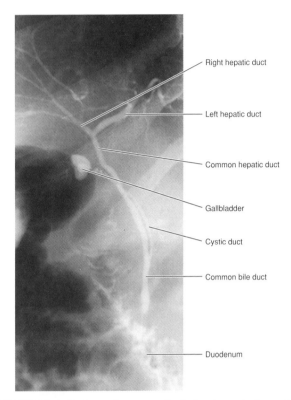

Right hepatic duct

Left hepatic duct

Common hepatic duct

Gallbladder

Cystic duct

Common bile duct

Duodenum

FIGURE 2-5. Endoscopic retrograde cholangiograph shows the normal gallbladder and biliary tree. Note that the cystic duct normally lies on the right side of the common hepatic duct and joins it superior to the duodenal cap. (From Dudek RW, Louis TM. *High-Yield Gross Anatomy.* 3rd ed. Baltimore: Lippincott Williams & Wilkins; 2008:125.)

Clinical Significance

Gall Stones

Concretions (gall stones) from the gall bladder may lodge in the hepatopancreatic ampulla, causing bile to backup into the pancreas, leading to pancreatitis, jaundice, and pain. The gall bladder is often removed via laparoscopic cholecystectomy.

Vessels of the gall bladder
(Figures 2-3 and 2-4)

Artery	Origin	Description
Celiac trunk	Abdominal aorta	Gives rise to splenic, hepatic, and left gastric arteries; supplies embryologic foregut
Hepatic	Celiac trunk	Gives rise to right and left hepatic arteries
Right and left hepatic arteries	Hepatic	Gives rise to cystic
Cystic	Right hepatic	Supplies gall bladder and cystic duct

Additional Concept

Venous Drainage

Venous drainage from the biliary tree and neck of the gall bladder is via the cystic veins—they either drain directly into the liver or into the portal vein. Venous drainage from the remainder of the gall bladder is directly into the liver.

Nerves of the gall bladder

Nerve	Origin	Structures Innervated
Parasympathetic	Vagal	Presynaptic parasympathetic fibers synapse on nerve cell bodies in the wall of the gall bladder
Sympathetic	Presynaptics originate in the intermediolateral cell column of the spinal cord and travel in the sympathetic trunks and splanchnic nerves to reach abdominal plexuses	Postsynaptic fibers travel on branches of arteries to reach the gall bladder
Visceral afferent	Cell bodies located in spinal ganglia	Gall bladder sensitive to pain
Right phrenic		• Somatic afferent innervation, primarily mediating pain • Conveyed to cervical spinal cord

PANCREAS

Structure of the pancreas
(Figures 2-3 and 2-5)

The pancreas is an elongated, lobulated, retroperitoneal organ found along the posterior abdominal wall. It has both an exocrine and endocrine function:

- exocrine—produces pancreatic digestive enzymes
- endocrine—produces glucagon and insulin

Structure	Description	Significance
Parts		
Head	Expanded part	Lies in concavity of the C-shaped duodenum
Uncinate process	Hook-shaped projection from head	• Posterior relations: inferior vena cava, right renal vessels and left renal vein • Anterior relations: superior mesenteric artery
Neck	Short part between head and body	Overlies junction of superior mesenteric and splenic veins to form the portal vein
Body	Part between neck and tail	Lies to the left of the superior mesenteric vessels
Tail	• Mobile • Located in splenorenal ligament	Related to hilum of spleen and left colic flexure
Features		
Main pancreatic duct	• Begins at tail and extends to head • Conveys pancreatic enzymes • Release of pancreatic enzymes regulated by smooth muscle sphincter—**sphincter of pancreatic duct**	• Merges with bile duct in head of pancreas to form **hepatopancreatic ampulla,** which opens into descending part of duodenum at the **major duodenal papilla** • Release of contents into the duodenum is controlled by a smooth muscle sphincter—**hepatopancreatic sphincter** (sphincter of Oddi) that surrounds the ampulla
Accessory pancreatic duct	• Drains uncinate process and part of head of pancreas • Conveys pancreatic enzymes	Empties into descending part of duodenum at **minor duodenal papilla**

The remainder of the biliary tree is presented with the gall bladder and liver.

Clinical Significance

Pancreatic Cancer

Pancreatic cancer results in a low survival rate as a result of difficulty to identify and treat because of its location and easy route of metastasis to the liver.

Vessels of the pancreas
(Figures 2-3 and 2-4)

Artery	Origin	Description
Celiac trunk	Abdominal aorta	• Gives rise to splenic, hepatic, and left gastric arteries • Supplies embryologic foregut
Splenic	Celiac trunk	Gives rise to dorsal, caudal, and great pancreatic arteries
Dorsal pancreatic	Splenic	Supplies body and tail
Great pancreatic		
Caudal pancreatic		
Hepatic	Celiac	Gives rise to gastroduodenal
Gastroduodenal	Hepatic	Gives rise to anterior and posterior superior pancreaticoduodenals
Anterior and posterior superior pancreaticoduodenals	Gastroduodenal	Supply head and neck
Superior mesenteric	Abdominal aorta	• Gives rise to anterior and posterior inferior pancreaticoduodenals • Supplies alimentary canal to left colic flexure • Supplies embryologic midgut
Anterior and posterior inferior pancreaticoduodenals	Superior mesenteric	Supply head and neck

Additional Concept

Venous Drainage

Venous drainage is via the splenic and superior mesenteric veins, which join to form the portal vein.

Nerves of the pancreas

Nerve	Origin	Structures Innervated
Parasympathetic	Vagus nerves	• Anterior and posterior vagal trunks enter abdomen through the esophageal hiatus • Secretomotor, although most pancreatic secretion is controlled hormonally
Sympathetic	Presynaptics originate from the intermediolateral cell column of the spinal cord and travel in the sympathetic trunks splanchnic nerves to reach abdominal plexuses	• Presynaptic sympathetics are conveyed to the celiac and superior mesenteric plexuses • Postsynaptic fibers travel on branches of celiac and superior mesenteric arteries to pancreas • Most pancreatic secretion is controlled hormonally

SPLEEN

Structure of the spleen
(Figure 2-3)

The spleen is a lymphatic organ located in the upper left quadrant of the abdomen. It functions to remove old or abnormal red blood cells, stores platelets, and produces antibodies.

Structure	Description	Significance
Hilum	Medially directed concavity	• Site of entry and exit to and from the spleen • Tail of the pancreas contacts spleen here
Gastrosplenic ligament	Connects hilum of spleen to greater curvature of stomach	• Part of greater omentum • Contains short gastric and left gastroepiploic vessels
Splenorenal ligament	Connects hilum of spleen to left kidney	• Double layer of peritoneum • Contains splenic vessels

Clinical Significance

Splenomegaly

The spleen may enlarge (splenomegaly) from a variety of reasons or may be damaged by broken ribs, causing profuse bleeding.

Vessels of the spleen
(Figures 2-3 and 2-4)

Artery	Origin	Description
Celiac trunk	Abdominal aorta	• Gives rise to splenic, hepatic, and left gastric arteries • Supplies embryologic foregut
Splenic	Celiac trunk	• Easily identified by tortuous course • Travels in splenorenal ligament • Supplies spleen via 5 terminal branches

Additional Concept

Venous Drainage

Venous drainage is via the splenic vein, which joins the superior mesenteric vein to form the portal vein.

Nerves of the spleen

Nerve	Origin	Structures Innervated
Parasympathetic	Vagus nerves	Anterior and posterior vagal trunks enter abdomen through the esophageal hiatus
Sympathetic	Presynaptics originate from the intermediolateral cell column of the spinal cord and travel in the sympathetic trunks and splanchnic nerves to reach abdominal plexuses	• Presynaptic sympathetics are conveyed to the celiac plexus/ganglia • Postsynaptic fibers travel on branches of the splenic artery to the spleen

KIDNEYS

Structure of the kidneys
(Figures 2-6 and 2-7)

The kidneys and ureters are retroperitoneal organs located along the posterior abdominal wall. The kidneys function to remove excess water, salts, and wastes from the blood. The ureters convey urine from the kidney to the urinary bladder.

Structure of the kidneys *(continued)*

Structure	Description	Significance
Parts		
Renal capsule	Thin connective tissue capsule that surrounds kidney	• Outer surface of kidney • Surrounded by perirenal fat
Renal cortex	• Between renal capsule and renal medulla • Extends into renal medulla as renal columns	Consists of cortical labyrinth and cortical rays
Renal medulla	Between renal cortex and renal hilum	Contains renal pyramids and renal columns
Renal hilum	Concave medial-margin of kidney	Bounds renal sinus
Renal pyramid	• 5–10; conical-shaped • Base adjacent to cortex, apex forms renal papilla	• Compose major part of medulla • Renal columns intervene between adjacent pyramids
Renal papilla	• 5–10 • Tip of renal pyramid	Open into minor calyces
Renal sinus	Area bounded by renal hilum	• Space in concave medial-margin of kidney • Contains renal vein, renal artery, and renal pelvis from anterior to posterior
Minor calyces	Located in renal sinus; convey urine	Several minor calyces merge to form major calyces
Major calyces		• Formed by merging of several minor calyces • Several major calyces merge to form renal pelvis
Renal pelvis	• Located in renal sinus • Proximal expanded end of ureter • Formed by merging of major calyces	Narrows to form **ureter**— • Retroperitoneal • Conveys urine from kidney to urinary bladder
Features		
Perirenal fat	Layer of protective fat surrounding kidney and suprarenal glands	Continuous with fat in renal sinus
Renal fascia	Membranous layer between peri- and pararenal fat	• Surrounds kidney, suprarenal gland, and perirenal fat • Continuous with fascia on inferior aspect of diaphragm
Pararenal fat	Fat external to renal fascia	Thick, protective layer of fat

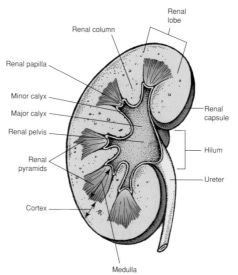

FIGURE 2-6. Longitudinal section of the kidney, near the hilum. (From *Stedman's Medical Dictionary.* 27th ed. Baltimore: Lippincott Williams & Wilkins; 2000.)

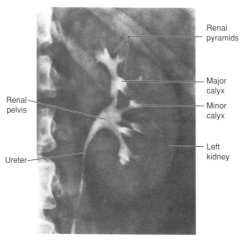

FIGURE 2-7. Intravenous urogram showing left kidney and proximal ureter; note the calyces and renal pelvis. (From Dudek RW, Louis TM. *High-Yield Gross Anatomy.* 3rd ed. Baltimore: Lippincott Williams & Wilkins; 2008:164.)

Clinical Significance

Constrictions of the Ureters

Ureters are constricted at three places: (1) at the junction with the renal pelvis; (2) where they cross the pelvic brim; and (3) as they pass through the wall of the urinary bladder.

Kidney Transplantation

Kidney transplantation is a well-established procedure to replace failing kidneys. The transplanted kidney is placed in the iliac fossa (of the pelvis) for support.

Kidney Stones

Kidney stones (renal calculi) are concretions that form in the kidneys and may lodge in the calices, ureters, or urinary bladder. Kidney stones may block urine passage and cause pain referred to nearby regions.

Vessels of the kidneys and ureters

Artery	Origin	Description
Right and left renal	Abdominal aorta	• Gives rise to 4–5 segmental arteries • Supply superior aspect of ureter
Segmental (4–5)	Renal arteries	Supply segments of the kidney
Right and left gonadal (testicular or ovarian)	Abdominal aorta	Supply middle aspects of ureter
Abdominal aorta	Continuous with thoracic aorta	Supply inferior aspects of ureter
Vein	**Termination**	**Description**
Renal	Inferior vena cava	Drain kidneys and ureters
Gonadal	• Right gonadal terminates in inferior vena cava • Left gonadal terminates in left renal vein	Drain ureters

Nerves of the kidneys and ureters

Nerve	Origin	Structures Innervated
Sympathetic	Presynaptics originate intermediolateral cell column of the spinal cord travel in sympathetic trunks and splanchnic nerves to reach abdominal plexuses	• Presynaptic sympathetics are conveyed to the renal, abdominal aortic and superior hypogastric plexuses/ganglia • Postsynaptic fibers travel on arterial branches to kidney and ureter; regulate blood pressure by effecting renin release
Visceral afferent	Cell bodies located in spinal ganglia	Mediate pain sensation

Additional Concept

Parasympathetic Innervation

Parasympathetic innervation of the kidneys is negligible. Autonomic innervation of the ureters is modulatory, but not necessary to maintain the peristaltic contractions that convey urine to the bladder.

SUPRARENAL GLANDS

Structure of the suprarenal glands

The suprarenal glands are positioned between the kidneys and crura of the diaphragm. The right gland is pyramidal-shaped, whereas the left is crescent-shaped. They are surrounded by perirenal fat and renal fascia and separated from the kidney connective tissue. The suprarenal glands function to secrete hormones and norepinephrine and epinephrine.

Structure	Description	Significance
Cortex	Outer part	Secretes corticosteroids and androgens
Medulla	Inner part	• Secretes norepinephrine and epinephrine • Composed of modified postsynaptic sympathetic neurons

Vessels of the suprarenal glands
(Figure 2-4)

Artery	Origin	Description
Inferior phrenic	Abdominal aorta	Gives rise to superior suprarenal
Superior suprarenal	Inferior phrenic	Part of rich blood supply to gland
Middle suprarenal	Abdominal aorta	
Renal		Gives rise to inferior suprarenal
Inferior suprarenal	Renal	Part of rich blood supply to gland
Vein	**Termination**	**Description**
Right suprarenal	Inferior vena cava	Drain gland
Left suprarenal	Left renal	

Nerves of the suprarenal glands

Nerve	Origin	Structures innervated
Sympathetic	Presynaptics originate from the intermediolateral cell column of the spinal cord and travel in the sympathetic trunks and splanchnic nerves to reach abdominal plexuses	Presynaptic sympathetics are conveyed to the suprarenal glands by traveling on arterial branches, where they synapse on cells of the medulla

ABDOMINAL LYMPHATICS

Abdominal lymphatics

Structure	Description	Drainage
Abdominal wall	Superficial lymphatic vessels accompany subcutaneous veins	• Superior to umbilicus—drain to axillary nodes • Inferior to umbilicus—drain to superficial inguinal nodes
Esophagus	Into left gastric lymph nodes	Left gastric nodes drain into celiac nodes
Stomach	Vessels accompany arteries along curvatures of stomach	Lymph is collected in gastric and gastro-omental nodes, which drain into pancreaticosplenic, pyloric, and pancreaticoduodenal lymph nodes, all of which eventually drain to the celiac nodes

(continued)

Abdominal lymphatics *(continued)*

Structure	Description	Drainage
Small intestine	• Duodenum: vessels accompany arteries • Jejunum and ileum: drainage begins as specialized vessels—lacteals in the intestinal villi	• Duodenum: anterior vessels drain into pancreaticoduodenal nodes, which drain into pyloric nodes; posterior vessels drain into superior mesenteric nodes, all of which eventually drain into celiac nodes • Jejunum and ileum: lacteals form vessels that drain into juxta-intestinal nodes to mesenteric nodes to superior central nodes, all of which eventually drain into superior mesenteric lymph nodes that drain to the ileocolic nodes
Large intestine	• Cecum and appendix: vessels to the nodes in the mesoappendix and ileocolic lymph nodes • Ascending, descending, and sigmoid colon: vessels to epicolic and paracolic nodes • Transverse colon: vessels to middle colic nodes • Rectum: superior half: drain to pararectal nodes; inferior half: drain to sacral nodes • Anal canal: superior to pectinate line: drain to internal iliac nodes; inferior to pectinate line: drain to superficial inguinal nodes	• Cecum and appendix: nodes in the mesoappendix and ileocolic nodes drain to the superior mesenteric nodes • Ascending, descending, and sigmoid colon: epiploic and paracolic nodes drain to ileocolic and right colic nodes, which drain to superior mesenteric lymph nodes • Transverse colon: middle colic nodes drain to superior mesenteric nodes • Rectum: pararectal nodes drain to inferior mesenteric nodes, sacral nodes follow middle rectal vessels to internal iliac nodes • Anal canal: internal iliac nodes drain to the common iliac and eventually the lumbar lymph nodes; superficial inguinal nodes drain to the deep inguinal lymph nodes
Spleen	Vessels follow arteries from the hilum	Vessels lead to pancreaticosplenic nodes, which lead to superior mesenteric lymph nodes

(continued)

Abdominal lymphatics *(continued)*

Structure	Description	Drainage
Pancreas	Vessels follow arteries	Vessels lead to pancreatico-splenic nodes and pyloric nodes, which lead to the superior mesenteric lymph nodes
Suprarenal glands		Drain to lumbar lymph nodes
Kidney and ureter	Kidney and superior aspect of ureter: vessels follow arteries	• Kidney and superior aspect of ureter: drain to the lumbar nodes • Mid-ureter: drain to common iliac nodes • Inferior ureter lymph is conveyed to iliac lymph nodes
Gall bladder	Lymphatics are first conveyed to the hepatic nodes	Lymph from hepatic nodes is conveyed to celiac nodes
Liver	Efferent lymphatics drain to the hepatic nodes (deep lymphatics), to phrenic nodes (superficial lymphatics) or posterior mediastinal nodes	• Produces ~50% of the lymph conveyed by the **thoracic duct** • Most lymph from the liver is conveyed to the **cisterna chyli**—the dilated beginning of the thoracic duct

Additional Concept

Thoracic Duct

The **thoracic duct** begins in the abdomen as the **cisterna chyli** and conveys lymph from both lower limbs, the entire abdomen, the left half of the thoracic cavity via a thoracic trunk, the left upper limb via a subclavian trunk, and left side of the head and neck via the jugular trunk to the junction of the subclavian and internal jugular veins.

Right Lymphatic Duct

The **right lymphatic duct** conveys lymph from the remainder of the body (right side of thorax via a thoracic trunk, right upper limb via a subclavian trunk, right side of head and neck via a jugular trunk) to the junction of the internal jugular and subclavian veins on the right.

Lymphatic vessels associated with abdominal viscera generally follow vessels (arteries) and are conveyed to lumbar and intestinal lymphatic vessels/trunks, which lead to the cisterna chyli.

▨ INTRODUCTION

The pelvic cavity is the inferior portion of the abdomino-pelvic cavity and as such has many features and structures in common with the abdominal cavity; many organs and peritoneal relations are continuous between the two. The pelvic cavity contains parts of the urinary system and the internal genitals.

The perineum is the area between the thighs and the location of the external genitalia in both sexes.

PELVIS

Areas of the pelvis

The pelvic cavity is continuous superiorly with the abdominal cavity.

Area	Structure	Significance
Pelvic inlet (superior pelvic aperture)	Bounded by: • Pubic symphysis and crest • Pectineal line • Arcuate line of the ilium and the ala of each side • Promontory of the sacrum	Collectively the structures that bound the pelvic inlet are known as the **linea terminalis** or **pelvic brim**
Pelvic outlet	Bounded by: • Pubic symphysis • Ischiopubic ramus and ischial tuberosity • Sacrotuberous ligaments • Coccyx	In the female, the pelvic outlet is larger than in the male to accommodate parturition

(continued)

Areas of the pelvis *(continued)*

Area	Structure	Significance
Greater pelvis (false pelvis)	Bounded by: • Lateral—ala of the ilium • Inferior—pelvic inlet • Superior—continuous with abdominal cavity • Anterior—abdominal wall • Posterior—L5–S1 vertebrae	• Superior aspect of the pelvis • Contains abdominal viscera, including the sigmoid colon and parts of the ileum
Lesser pelvis (true pelvis)	Bounded by: • Superior—pelvic inlet (superior pelvic aperture) • Inferior—pelvic outlet and pelvic diaphragm • Lateral—hip bones • Posterior—sacrum and coccyx • Anterior—pubic symphysis	• Inferior aspect of the pelvis • Contains reproductive and urinary organs, including the urinary bladder, uterus (female), and prostate (male)
Retropubic space	Potential, fat-filled area of endopelvic fascia between the pubic symphysis and urinary bladder	Allows for the expansion of the urinary bladder as it fills with urine
Retrorectal space	Potential, fat-filled area of endopelvic fascia between the rectum and sacrum and coccyx	Allows for the expansion of the rectum during defecation

Clinical Significance

Pregnancy

The size of the lesser pelvis increases and the pubic symphysis becomes more flexible in pregnant females as hormones cause the pelvic ligaments to relax.

Bones of the pelvis
(Figure 3-1)

Feature	Characteristic	Significance
Pelvic girdle	Basin-shaped group of bones: 2 hip bones and the sacrum	• Transfers weight from vertebral column to lower limbs

(continued)

Bones of the pelvis *(continued)*

Feature	Characteristic	Significance
		• Hip bones joined anteriorly by **pubic symphysis,** joined to sacrum posteriorly at sacroiliac joints
Greater sciatic foramen	Sacrospinous ligament forms greater sciatic notch into foramen	Permits passage of piriformis, gluteal vessels, and nerves, sciatic and posterior femoral cutaneous nerves, internal pudendal vessels, pudendal nerve, and nerves to obturator internus and quadratus femoris from the pelvis to the gluteal region
Lesser sciatic foramen	Sacrospinous and sacrotuberous ligaments form foramen	Permits passage of the tendon of obturator internus and the internal pudendal vessels and pudendal nerve as they wrap around the ischial spine to enter the perineum
Obturator foramen	Formed by body and ramus of ischium and superior and inferior pubic rami	• Covered by obturator membrane • A deficiency in the obturator membrane—the **obturator canal:** permits passage of obturator vessels and nerves between the pelvis and lower limb
Acetabulum	• Formed by contributions from the ilium, ischium, and pubis • Deficient inferiorly as the **acetabular notch**	• Cup-shaped articular cavity on lateral aspect of hip bone • Head of femur articulates here • Acetabular notch bridged by **transverse acetabular ligament** to complete cup
Pubic arch	Formed by both ischiopubic rami, which meet at the pubic symphysis	Inferior borders of ischiopubic rami form **subpubic angle,** which is typically <70° in males and >80° in females
Hip Bones—formed by the fusion of the ilium, ischium, and pubis		
Ilium	Ala	• Expanded upper portion of ilium • Superior border is the **iliac crest** • Posterior gluteal surface bears 3 lines: the **anterior, middle,**

(continued)

Bones of the pelvis *(continued)*

Feature	Description	Significance
		and **posterior gluteal lines** that serve as attachments for muscles of the gluteal region • Anterior surface—iliac fossa
	Body	• The smaller inferior portion of the ilium • Forms part of acetabulum
	Arcuate line	• Junction of the body of the ilium and body of the ischium • Part of linea terminalis
	Iliac crest	• Superior border of ala • Attachment for abdominal, back, and lower limb muscles • Located between the anterior and posterior superior iliac spines
	Anterior superior iliac spine	• Anterior end of iliac crest • Attachment for fascia lata, tensor of fascia lata, sartorius, and inguinal ligament
	Posterior superior iliac spine	• Posterior end of iliac crest • Attachment for multifidus • Site of skin dimples • Marks S2 vertebral level and inferior end of dural sac
	Anterior inferior iliac spine	Attachment for rectus femoris
	Posterior inferior iliac spine	Superior border of greater sciatic notch
	Iliac fossa	• Depression on anterior aspect of ala • Proximal attachment for iliacus
	Greater sciatic notch	Between posterior inferior iliac spine and ischial spine
Ischium	Body	• Forms part of acetabulum • Ischial spine and tuberosity project from body
	Ramus	Articulates with inferior ramus of pubis
	Ischial tuberosity	• Projection from body of ischium • Attachment for adductor magnus, the hamstrings, and the sacrotuberous ligament

(continued)

Bones of the pelvis *(continued)*

Feature	Description	Significance
	Ischial spine	• Projection from body • Attachment for superior gemellus, coccygeus, levator ani, and **sacrospinous ligament**—which converts the greater sciatic notch into a foramen • Forms superior border of lesser sciatic notch
Pubis	Body	Forms part of acetabulum
	Superior ramus	• Articulates with contralateral superior ramus • Pubic tubercle projects from superior ramus • Contributes to obturator foramen
	Pubic tubercle	• Projection from superior ramus • Attachment for inguinal ligament and inferior crus of superficial inguinal ring
	Pectin pubis	• Ridge along superior ramus extending laterally from pubic tubercle • Attachment for lacunar ligament and conjoint tendon
	Inferior ramus	Contributes to obturator foramen

The gluteal-aspect (posterior) of the bones in this table is described with the skeletal sections of the lower limb and back.

Additional Concept

Greater Sciatic Foramen

The **greater sciatic foramen** is considered an exit from the pelvis. Of the structures passing out of the pelvis via the foramen, only the superior gluteal vessels and nerves pass superior to the piriformis, all other structures pass inferior to this landmark muscle.

Ischiopubic Ramus

The **ramus** of the ischium and the **inferior ramus** of the pubis are collectively known as the **ischiopubic ramus**.

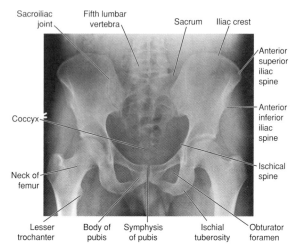

FIGURE 3-1. Bones of the pelvis radiograph. (From Dudek RW, Louis TM. *High-Yield Gross Anatomy.* 3rd ed. Baltimore: Lippincott Williams & Wilkins; 2008:211.)

Clinical Significance

Sex Differences in the Pelves

The pelves differ between the sexes: the female pelvis is specialized for parturition. The female pelvis is lightweight, wide, and shallow, with an oval pelvic inlet and larger pelvic outlet and subpubic angle relative to the male pelvis.

Minimum diameters of the pelvis are important in obstetrics. The obstetric "true" conjugate—the distance between the posterior aspect of the pubic symphysis and the sacral promontory should be >11 cm for vaginal delivery.

Joints of the pelvis
(Figure 3-1)

Joint	Type	Articulation	Structure
Sacroiliac	• Anterior part: synovial	Sacrum suspended between iliac bones	• Joint strengthened by anterior, posterior, and interosseous **sacroiliac ligaments**

(continued)

Joints of the pelvis *(continued)*

Joint	Type	Articulation	Structure
	• Posterior part: fibrous		• **Sacrotuberous** and **sacrospinous ligaments** provide resilient support during times of sudden weight increases (e.g., jumping)
Pubic symphysis	Cartilaginous	Between bodies of pubic bones	• Interpubic disc located between bones • Joint strengthened by superior and inferior pubic ligaments; also strengthened by tendons of rectus abdominis and external oblique

The joints associated with the vertebral column are described with the back (see Chapter 4).

Peritoneum of the pelvis
(Figure 3-6)

The peritoneum lining the greater sac of the abdomen continues into the pelvis; it reflects onto the organs of the pelvis creating pouches and fossae.

Feature	Description	Significance
Female		
Supravesical fossa	Between anterior abdominal wall and urinary bladder	Reflection of peritoneum from anterior abdominal wall onto superior surface of urinary bladder • Allows for expansion of urinary bladder
Vesicouterine pouch	Between urinary bladder and uterus	• Reflection of peritoneum from urinary bladder onto uterus • Allows for expansion of uterus and urinary bladder • Potential site for fluid accumulation during pathologic processes
Rectouterine pouch	Between uterus and rectum	• Reflection of peritoneum from uterus to rectum

(continued)

Peritoneum of the pelvis *(continued)*

Feature	Description	Significance
		• Allows for expansion of rectum and uterus • Potential site for fluid accumulation during pathologic processes
Male		
Supravesical fossa	Between anterior abdominal wall and urinary bladder	Reflection of peritoneum from anterior abdominal wall onto superior surface of urinary bladder • Allows for expansion of urinary bladder
Rectovesical pouch	Between urinary bladder and rectum	• Reflection of peritoneum from urinary bladder onto rectum • Allows for expansion of rectum and urinary bladder • Potential site for fluid accumulation during pathologic processes

Fascia of the pelvis
(Figure 3-6)

Fascia/Connective Tissue	Significance/Structure
Pelvic fascia	• Inferior continuation of endoabdominal fascia • Between parietal peritoneum and muscular body wall
Parietal layer of pelvic fascia	Membranous layer of pelvic fascia that lines the muscles of the pelvic walls
Visceral layer of pelvic fascia	Membranous layer of pelvic fascia that invests the organs of the pelvis as their adventitial layer
Tendinous arch of pelvic fascia	Anteroposterior oriented bilateral thickening of pelvic fascia formed at points of reflection between the parietal and visceral layers of pelvic fascia (just lateral to where organs penetrate pelvic floor)
Puboprostatic ligament	Anterior subdivision of tendinous arch in the male that connects the prostate to the pubis
Pubovesical ligament	Anterior subdivision of tendinous arch in the female that connects the neck of the bladder to the pubis
Endopelvic fascia	Layer of fascia connecting the visceral and parietal layers of pelvic fascia of varying consistency

(continued)

Fascia of the pelvis *(continued)*

Fascia/Connective Tissue	Significance/Structure
Transverse cervical (cardinal) ligament	• Condensed layer of endopelvic fascia in the female that provides the primary support for the uterus • Connects lateral wall of pelvis with the cervix of the uterus
Rectovesical septum	Condensed layer of endopelvic fascia in the male between the bladder and prostate and the rectum
Prostatic sheath	• Formed by the visceral layer of pelvic fascia • Surrounds fibrous capsule of the prostate • Continuous anteriorly with the puboprostatic ligaments and posteriorly with the rectovesical septum

Muscles of the pelvis
(Figures 3-2, 3-3, and 3-6)

Muscle	Proximal Attachment	Distal Attachment	Innervation	Main Actions
Obturator internus	Obturator membrane, ilium, and ischium	Greater trochanter of femur	Nerve to obturator internus (L5–S2)	Laterally rotates thigh, holds femur in acetabulum
Piriformis	Sacrum (S2–S4 segments), sacrotuberous ligament, margin of greater sciatic notch		S1–S2	Laterally rotates and abducts thigh; holds femur in acetabulum
Levator ani (iliococcygeus, pubococcygeus [largest part] and puborectalis)	Pubis, tendinous arch of obturator internus and ischial spine	Perineal body, coccyx, anococcygeal ligament, walls of prostate, vagina, rectum and anal canal	Pudendal and nerve to levator ani	• Part of pelvic diaphragm • Supports pelvic viscera • Puborectalis part forms sling around **anorectal junction**—responsible for fecal continence
Coccygeus	Ischial spine	Sacrum and coccyx	S4–S5	Part of pelvic diaphragm • Supports pelvic viscera

Additional Concept

Pelvic Diaphragm

The **pelvic diaphragm** is the funnel-shaped floor of the pelvis, formed by the **levator ani** and **coccygeus**. The levator ani is subdivided based on attachment into iliococcygeus, pubococcygeus, and puborectalis from superior to inferior.

Obturator Fascia

A thickening of the fascia of the obturator internus—the **obturator fascia** on the medial surface of the muscle—forms the **tendinous arch of levator ani**, which serves as an attachment for levator ani.

Sacral Plexus

The **sacral plexus** sits on the muscular "bed" of the **piriformis**.

Clinical Significance

Trauma to the Pelvic Floor

The muscles forming the floor of the pelvis may be injured during childbirth. Trauma to the pubococcygeus, the main part of the levator ani or the nerves supplying it, may lead to urinary incontinence.

Nerves of the pelvis
(Figures 3-2, 3-3, and 3-6)

The lumbosacral trunk conveys fibers from the L4–L5 spinal cord levels to the sacral plexus (S1–S4). The sacral plexus innervates pelvic structures, the perineum, and the lower limb; it is formed of anterior rami.

Nerve	Origin	Structures Innervated
Sacral Plexus		
Sciatic	L4–S3	Supplies hip joint, leg, foot and posterior compartment of the thigh
Pudendal	S2–S4	• Supplies perineal musculature, sphincter urethrae, and external anal sphincter • Sensory to skin covering external genitalia
Superior gluteal	L4–S1	Supplies gluteus medius and minimus and tensor of fascia lata
Inferior gluteal	L5–S2	Supplies gluteus maximus

(continued)

Nerve	Origin	Structures Innervated
Nerve to piriformis	S1–S2	Supplies piriformis
Nerve to quadratus femoris	L4–S1	Supplies quadratus femoris and inferior gemellus
Nerve to obturator internus	L5–S2	Supplies obturator internus and superior gemellus
Nerve to levator ani	S3–S4	Supplies levator ani and coccygeus
Posterior femoral cutaneous	S2–S3	Sensory to inferior aspect of buttock and posterior aspect of thigh
Coccygeal Plexus—sparse fibers from lower sacral and coccygeal spinal cord levels that inconsistently provide sensory and motor innervation to nearby regions and structures.		
Autonomic Innervation of the Pelvis		
Sympathetic	Sacral levels of the sympathetic trunks convey postsynaptic sympathetic fibers, and sacral splanchnic nerves to plexuses in the pelvis	Fibers join the hypogastric, pelvic, sacral, and coccygeal plexuses and follow arteries to their targets—arteries, urinary bladder, prostate, seminal glands, uterus, vagina, and genitals
Parasympathetic	S2–S4 contain presynaptic parasympathetic fibers that are conveyed via pelvic splanchnic nerves to plexuses in the pelvis	Fibers join the hypogastric and pelvic plexuses and follow arteries to their targets—urinary bladder, rectum, and genitals, where they synapse in the wall of the organ
Visceral afferents	Inferior to pelvic pain line: convey sensation to S2–S4 levels via pelvic splanchnics; superior to pelvic pain line: convey sensation to thoracic and lumbar spinal cord levels	The **pelvic pain line** is indicated by the peritoneum as it drapes into the pelvis—structures in contact with the peritoneum are above the pain line; structures inferior to the peritoneum are below the pain line

Clinical Significance

Compression of the Sacral Plexus

The fetal head may compress branches of the sacral plexus during pregnancy and childbirth, producing pain in the lower limbs and back.

Mnemonic

Pudendal Nerve Roots

Pudendal and parasympathetic spinal cord levels: S2, S3, and S4 keep the genitals off the floor.

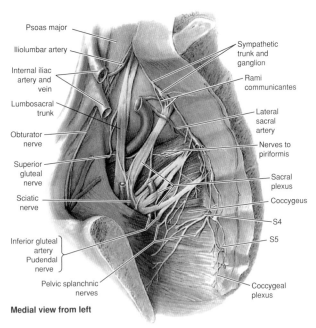

Psoas major
Iliolumbar artery
Internal iliac artery and vein
Lumbosacral trunk
Obturator nerve
Superior gluteal nerve
Sciatic nerve
Inferior gluteal artery
Pudendal nerve
Pelvic splanchnic nerves
Sympathetic trunk and ganglion
Rami communicantes
Lateral sacral artery
Nerves to piriformis
Sacral plexus
Coccygeus
S4
S5
Coccygeal plexus

Medial view from left

FIGURE 3-2. Nerves of the pelvis. Somatic nerves (sacral and coccygeal nerve plexuses) and the pelvic (sacral) part of the sympathetic trunk are shown. Although located in the pelvis, most of the nerves seen here are involved with the innervation of the lower limb rather than the pelvic structures. (From Moore KL, Dalley AF. *Clinically Oriented Anatomy.* 5th ed. Baltimore: Lippincott Williams & Wilkins; 2006:380.)

Vasculature of the pelvis
(Figures 3-2, 3-3, 3-4, and 3-6)

Artery	Origin	Description
Internal iliac	Common iliac	Supplies pelvis, gluteal region, thigh, and perineum
Anterior division	Internal iliac	Supplies pelvic viscera and medial compartment of the thigh
Posterior division		Supplies walls of pelvis and gluteal region
Umbilical	Anterior division	• Gives rise to superior vesical and occasionally uterine and vaginal arteries • Obliterated distal part forms medial umbilical ligaments
Obturator		Supplies superior aspect of medial compartment of thigh
Superior vesical	Umbilical	Supplies urinary bladder
Inferior vesical	Anterior division	Supplies urinary bladder, prostate, seminal gland, and ureter
Middle rectal		Supplies rectum, seminal gland, and prostate
Superior gluteal		Supplies superior aspect of gluteal region
Inferior gluteal		Supplies inferior aspect of gluteal region
Internal pudendal		Supplies perineum
Uterine/ vaginal		• May arise from anterior division or umbilical; may branch from common trunk • Supply uterus and vagina, respectively
Iliolumbar	Posterior division	Supplies iliacus, psoas, quadratus lumborum, and vertebral canal
Lateral sacral		Supplies piriformis and vertebral canal
Gonadal (testicular or ovarian)	Abdominal aorta	Supply testes and ovaries
Veins—veins draining to caval system generally follow arteries to terminate in the internal iliac vein; veins following portal system contribute to the inferior mesenteric vein		

Additional Concept

Venous Drainage

Venous drainage generally parallels arterial supply.

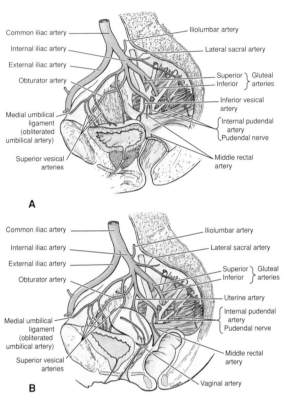

FIGURE 3-3. Arteries of the pelvis. The arteries of the male pelvis (**A**) and the female pelvis (**B**) are shown. Anterior divisions of the internal iliac arteries usually supply most of the blood to pelvic structures. The arteries are internal (lie medial) to the nerves making up the sacral plexus. (From Moore KL, Dalley AF. *Clinically Oriented Anatomy*. 5th ed. Baltimore: Lippincott Williams & Wilkins; 2006:386.)

Lymphatics of the pelvis

Structure	Description	Drainage
Urinary bladder	Vessels accompany	• Superior aspect: external iliac nodes • Inferior aspect: internal iliac nodes

(continued)

Lymphatics of the pelvis *(continued)*

Structure	Description	Drainage
Ureters	arteries—generally structures drain into external and internal iliac nodes, which drain into common iliac nodes to the lumbar nodes	Vessels drain to internal and external common iliac and lumbar nodes owing to their long course
Urethrae		• Male: vessels from prostatic and membranous portions drain to internal iliac nodes, whereas those from the penile urethra drain to the deep inguinal nodes • Female: vessels drain to the sacral and internal iliac nodes
Seminal glands		External and internal nodes
Prostate		Internal iliac and sacral nodes
Penis		Superficial and deep inguinal and external and internal iliac nodes
Vagina		• Superior aspect: internal and external iliac nodes • Middle aspect: internal iliac nodes • Inferior aspect: sacral and common iliac nodes • Drainage from the external vaginal orifice to superficial inguinal nodes
Uterus		• Fundus: lumbar nodes • Body: external iliac nodes • Cervix: internal iliac and sacral nodes
Ovaries		Lumbar nodes
Vulva		Superficial inguinal nodes

URINARY BLADDER

Structure of the urinary bladder
(Figures 3-3 and 3-6)

The bladder is a hollow, muscular organ that serves as reservoir for urine until it is voided. When empty, it is located entirely within the lesser pelvis; when full, it may extend through the extraperitoneal fascial plane superiorly as high as the umbilicus.

Structure	Description	Significance
Parts		
Body	Main part, between the apex and fundus	• In males—related to the rectum • In females—related to the vagina

(continued)

Structure of the urinary bladder *(continued)*

Structure	Description	Significance
Apex	Part directed toward the pubic symphysis	• Anterior-most aspect • Part from which the **urachus**—embryologic shunt for urine, originates
Neck	Inferior-most part	Anchored in place by the lateral ligaments of the bladder and the tendinous arch of pelvic fascia
Fundus	Convex, posteriorly-directed part	• Also known as the base • Location of the ureters as they enter the bladder
Features		
Detrusor muscle	• Composes the muscular part of the bladder wall • Internal wall covered with rugae to allow for expansion	Innervated by the parasympathetics S2–S4, causes constriction of wall and expulsion of urine
Internal urethral sphincter	Formed of circularly disposed smooth muscles fibers	• Located near neck of bladder • Contract during ejaculation to prevent semen from entering bladder
Internal urethral orifice	• Internal opening of the urethra • Located at inferior "corner" of urinary trigone	Radially arranged smooth muscle fibers assist in opening the sphincter to expel urine
Urinary trigone	Smooth inferoposterior aspect of bladder wall	3 corners of trigone: Inferior—internal urethral orifice and 2 superior—ureteric orifices

Additional Concept

Peritoneal Relations

The urinary bladder is covered only on its superior surface with peritoneum; the remainder is covered with loose connective tissue (vesical fascia). The bladder is relatively free except at the neck where it is held in place by the tendinous arch of the pelvis.

Median Umbilical Fold

The median umbilical ligament (vestige of the fetal urachus) is covered by peritoneum to form the median umbilical fold.

Vasculature of the urinary bladder

Artery	Origin	Description
Superior vesical	Umbilical	Supply anterior and superior aspects
Inferior vesical	Internal iliac	Males: supply posterior and inferior aspects
Vaginal	Uterine (sometimes via common trunk), umbilical, or internal iliac	Females: supply posterior and inferior aspects
Obturator	Internal iliac	May supply branches to bladder
Inferior gluteal		

Additional Concept

Venous Drainage

Venous drainage generally parallels arterial supply to end in the internal iliac vein.

Nerves of the urinary bladder

Nerve	Origin	Structures Innervated
Parasympathetic	S2–S4, conveyed via pelvic splanchnic nerves to pelvic plexuses	Motor to detrusor, inhibitory to internal urethral sphincter
Sympathetic	Presynaptics originate from the intermediolateral cell column of the spinal cord and travel in the sympathetic trunks and splanchnic nerves to reach pelvic plexuses	Motor to internal urethral sphincter
Visceral afferents	Bladder wall	• Senses stretching of bladder wall, impulses conveyed to spinal cord via pelvic splanchnics from most of bladder • Superior part of bladder is superior to pelvic pain line so impulses are conveyed via sympathetic system

URETHRAE

Structure of the urethrae
(Figures 3-3 and 3-6)

The urethrae extend from the internal urethral orifice of the urinary bladder to the external urethral orifice in both sexes. They function to convey urine from the urinary bladder to the outside world.

Structure	Description	Significance
Female urethra	• External urethral orifice located in the vestibule of the vagina • Passes through pelvic and urogenital (external urethral sphincter) diaphragms	• Located anterior to the vagina • Urethral glands open along length • Paraurethral glands open near external urethral orifice
Male urethra	• External urethral orifice located on tip of glans penis • Passes through pelvic and urogenital (external urethral sphincter) diaphragms	• Common route for urine and semen • Divided into 4 parts: 1. Intramural (preprostatic) 2. Prostatic 3. Membranous 4. Penile (spongy)

Clinical Significance

Catheterization

The short, distensible female urethra allows for easy passage of catheters into the bladder and provides an easy route for bacterial infection of the bladder.

Vasculature of the urethrae

Artery	Origin	Description
Female		
Internal pudendal	Anterior division of internal iliac	Supplies urethra and perineum
Vaginal		Supplies urethra and vagina
Male		
Inferior vesical	Anterior division of internal iliac	Supply intramural and prostatic parts via prostatic branches
Middle rectal		
Internal pudendal		Supplies membranous and penile parts

Additional Concept

Venous Drainage

Venous drainage generally parallels arterial supply.

Nerves of the urethrae

Nerve	Origin	Structures Innervated
Parasympathetic	Presynaptics originate in spinal cord levels S2–S4, conveyed via pelvic splanchnic nerves to pelvic plexuses	Inhibitory to internal urethral sphincter
Sympathetic	Presynaptics originate from the interomedio-lateral cell column of the spinal cord and travel in the sympathetic trunks and, finally, sacral splanchnic nerves to reach pelvic plexuses	Motor to internal urethral sphincter
Visceral afferents—both sexes	Urethra	Impulses conveyed to spinal cord via pelvic splanchnics
Somatic afferents—both sexes		Pain and general tactile impulses conveyed to spinal cord via pudendal nerve

FEMALE GENITALIA

Internal genitalia of the female
(Figures 3-3 and 3-4)

Structure	Description	Significance
Vagina		

Overall	• Extends from the uterus to the vaginal vestibule
	• Continuous superiorly with cervical canal at the **external os** of the uterus
	• **Vaginal fornices** (anterior, lateral, and posterior) surround uterine cervix
		• **Vaginal vestibule**—cleft between labia minora
		• Forms inferior part of birth canal, route for menses, and receives erect penis during copulation
		• Relations:
		  • Anterior—bladder
		  • Posterior—rectum
		  • Lateral—levator ani

(continued)

Internal genitalia of the female *(continued)*

Structure	Description	Significance
Vessels	• Arterial supply: uterine, vaginal, and internal pudendal • Venous drainage: via vaginal plexus to utero-vaginal venous plexus to internal iliac veins	Origin of arteries: anterior division of internal iliac
Innervation	• Motor: superior aspect—visceral, inferior aspect—somatic • Sensory: superior aspect—visceral, inferior aspect—somatic	• Visceral: uterovaginal nerve plexus contains sympathetics from the intermediolateral cell column, conveyed via the sympathetic chain and parasympathetics from S2–S4 spinal cord levels conveyed via pelvic splanchnics, visceral afferents travel with pelvic splanchnics • Somatic: pudendal nerve
Uterus		

Overall	• Structure:
	  • Fundus: superior to uterine tubes
	  • Body: main part, contains uterine cavity
	  • Isthmus: narrow region superior to cervix
	  • Cervix: possesses cervical canal with superior and inferior openings: the **internal** and **external os**
	• Relations:
	  • Anterior: bladder with intervening vesicouterine pouch
	  • Posterior: rectum with intervening rectouterine pouch
		• Thick-walled, muscular organ
		• Uterine cervix projects into superior aspect of vagina where it is surrounded by the vaginal fornices
		• The uterus is supported by ligaments (condensations of pelvic fascia) near the cervix—the transverse cervical (cardinal) and uterosacral ligaments

Vessels	• Arterial supply: uterine and ovarian • Venous drainage: via uterine plexus to uterovaginal plexus to internal iliac veins	Origin of arteries: anterior division of internal iliac

(continued)

Internal genitalia of the female *(continued)*

Structure	Description	Significance
Innervation	Innervation is from utero-vaginal plexus	Uterovaginal nerve plexus contains sympathetics from the intermediolateral cell column, conveyed via the sympathetic chain and parasympathetics from S2–S4 spinal cord levels conveyed via pelvic splanchnics, visceral afferents for pain travel with sympathetics above the pelvic pain line and with pelvic splanchnics below the pelvic pain line
Uterine Tubes		
Overall	• Bilateral; extend from the junction of the fundus and body of the uterus to open into the peritoneal cavity adjacent to the ovaries • Divided into infundibulum, ampulla, isthmus, and uterine parts	• Infundibulum—funnel-shaped end near ovary, possesses fimbriae: finger-like processes that envelope the medial pole of the ovary • Ampulla—longest part, normal site of fertilization • Isthmus—part that enters the uterus • Uterine part—intramural
Vessels	• Arterial supply: ovarian arteries • Venous drainage: empties into the ovarian veins and the uterovaginal venous plexus	Origin of arteries: abdominal aorta
Innervation	Innervation is from uterine and pelvic plexuses	Contain sympathetics from the intermediolateral cell column, conveyed via the sympathetic chain and parasympathetics from S2–S4 spinal cord levels conveyed via pelvic splanchnics, visceral afferents travel with sympathetics as the uterine tubes are above the pelvic pain line, some visceral afferents travel with pelvic splanchnics to mediate reflexes

(continued)

Internal genitalia of the female *(continued)*

Structure	Description	Significance
Ovaries		
Overall	• Located along lateral walls of pelvis • Held in relatively stable position by the **mesovarium, suspensory ligament of the ovary,** and the **ligament of the ovary**	• Not covered by peritoneum • The oocyte is ovulated into the peritoneal cavity • Fimbriae of the uterine tubes and the ciliated lining of the uterine tubes typically guide the oocyte into the ampulla of the uterine tube
Vessels	• Arterial supply: ovarian arteries • Venous drainage: small veins drain to a pampiniform venous plexus located within the broad ligament	• Origin: abdominal aorta • The **pampiniform plexus** of veins forms a pair of ovarian veins, the right ovarian vein empties into the inferior vena cava, whereas the left drains into the left renal vein
Innervation	Innervation is from uterine and pelvic plexuses	Contain sympathetics from the intermediolateral cell column, conveyed via the sympathetic chain and parasympathetics from S2–S4 spinal cord levels conveyed via pelvic splanchnics, visceral afferents travel with sympathetics as the uterine tubes are above the pelvic pain line, some visceral afferents travel with pelvic splanchnics to mediate reflexes

Additional Concept

Uterus

The uterus is typically anteverted (tipped anteriorly relative to the vagina) and anteflexed (body is flexed anteriorly relative to the cervix), but variations in degree and position are common.

The uterus is covered by peritoneum, which extends laterally off the uterus to the walls of the pelvis as the **broad ligament.** The broad ligament conveys uterine neurovascular elements between its layers and contains the ovaries and uterine tubes. The **suspensory ligament of the ovary** is a superolateral extension of the broad ligament from the ovary that conveys the ovarian vessels. The **ligament of the ovary** is found within the broad ligament and connects the ovary to the uterine body, whereas the **round ligament of the uterus**, also found within the broad ligament, projects from the uterine body through the inguinal canal to terminate as connective tissue septa in the labia majora. A posterior extension of broad ligament invests the ovary—the **mesovarium**, an extension of the broad ligament invests the uterine tube—the **mesosalpinx**. Inferior to the mesosalpinx the broad ligament is referred to as the **mesometrium**.

Embryologic Origins

The ligament of the ovary and the round ligament of the uterus are vestiges of the embryologic ovarian gubernaculums and are the equivalent of the very short scrotal ligament in the male.

External genitalia of the female
(Figure 3-4)

Structure	Description	Significance
Mons Pubis, Labia Major, and Labia Minora		
Overall	• Mons pubis and labia majora are prominent, fatty, pubic hair covered eminences surrounding the pudendal cleft • The labia minora are thin, fat-free folds of skin that enclose the vaginal vestibule	The labia minora are connected anteriorly, the posterior aspect of this connection forms the **frenulum of the clitoris,** whereas the anterior portion forms the **prepuce of the clitoris,** posteriorly they are united to form the **frenulum of the labia minora**
Vessels	• Arterial supply: labial branches • Venous drainage: parallels arterial supply	• Origin of arteries: internal pudendal • During sexual arousal—enlarge as a result of increased blood in underlying structures
Innervation	Pudendal	Pudendal and its branches (anterior and posterior labial) are chief source of sensory innervation

(continued)

External genitalia of the female *(continued)*

Structure	Description	Significance
Clitoris		
Overall	Parts: root and body; composed of 2 crura made of 2 erectile cylinders—the corpora cavernosa and **the glans of the clitoris**	• The **corpora cavernosa** diverge posteriorly to form crura that attach to ischiopubic rami for support and are invested by the ischiocavernosus muscles • The glans is the most sensitive part of the heavily innervated clitoris
Vessels	• Arterial supply: clitoral branches • Venous drainage: parallels arterial supply	• Origin of arteries: internal pudendal • Sexual arousal causes engorgement and enlargement from increased arterial supply and decreased venous return
Innervation	Pudendal and uterovaginal plexus	• Pudendal branches (dorsal nerve of the clitoris) provide somatic sensation • Parasympathetics from uterovaginal plexus cause erection
Bulbs of the Vestibule and Vestibular Glands		
Overall	• Bulbs of the vestibule are masses of erectile tissue underlying the labia majora • Vestibular glands lie posterior to the bulbs	• Bulbospongiosus invests the bulbs of the vestibule • The vestibular glands (greater and lesser) secrete mucus during sexual arousal to moisten the vestibule
Vessels	• Arterial supply: branches of the internal pudendal • Venous drainage parallels arterial supply	• Origin of arteries: internal pudendal • Sexual arousal causes engorgement and enlargement of the bulbs of the vestibule from increased arterial supply and decreased venous return
Innervation	Uterovaginal plexus	Parasympathetics from uterovaginal plexus cause erection and increased secretion from the glands

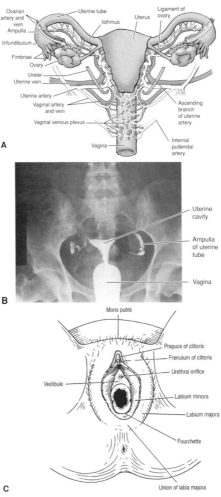

FIGURE 3-4. Female pelvis. **A:** Diagram of the arterial supply and venous drainage of the ovaries, uterine tubes, uterus, and vagina. **B:** Anteroposterior radiograph of the female pelvis after injection of a radiopaque compound into the uterine cavity (hysterosalpingography). **C:** Diagram of the female genitalia. (From Dudek RW, Louis TM. *High-Yield Gross Anatomy.* 3rd ed. Baltimore: Lippincott Williams & Wilkins; 2008:185.)

Additional Concept

Collectively, the external genitalia of the female are referred to as the **vulva** or pudendum. The labia majora enclose a space—**pudendal cleft**, which contain the labia minora and vaginal vestibule, whereas the labia minor enclose the **vaginal vestibule**, which contains the vaginal orifice, external urethral orifice (with openings of the ducts of the paraurethral glands on either side), and openings of the vestibular glands.

MALE GENITALIA

Internal genitalia of the male
(Figures 3-3 and 3-5)

Structure	Description	Significance
Ductus Deferens (2)		
Overall	Begins in scrotum at tail of epididymis; ends by joining duct of seminal gland to form **ejaculatory duct**	• Proximal continuation of epididymis • Ascends as part of spermatic cord; possesses an ampulla—an expansion near its distal end
Vessels	• Arterial supply: artery to the ductus deferens • Venous drainage parallels arteries	Origin of arteries: superior vesical artery
Innervation	Innervation is from the pelvic plexus	Contains sympathetics from the intermediolateral cell column, conveyed via the sympathetic chain and sacral splanchnics and parasympathetics from S2–S4 spinal cord levels conveyed via pelvic splanchnics
Seminal Glands		
Overall	• Located between urinary bladder and rectum—separated from it by the rectovesical pouch • Duct joins with ductus deferens to form ejaculatory duct	• Secrete a thick alkaline fluid that contributes to semen
Vessels	• Arterial supply: small branches • Venous drainage parallels arteries	Origin of arteries: inferior vesical and middle rectal

(continued)

Internal genitalia of the male (continued)

Structure	Description	Significance
Innervation	Innervation is from the pelvic plexus	Contains sympathetics from the intermediolateral cell column, conveyed via the sympathetic chain and parasympathetics from S2–S4 spinal cord levels conveyed via pelvic splanchnics
Ejaculatory Ducts		
Overall	Formed by the union of the ductus deferens and the duct of the seminal gland	• Open near the **prostatic utricle** in the prostatic urethra • Secrete fluid from the seminal gland and sperm from the ductus deferens
Vessels	• Arterial supply: artery to the ductus deferens • Venous drainage is to prostatic and vesical venous plexuses	Origin of arteries: superior (or inferior) vesical artery
Innervation	Innervation is from the pelvic plexus	Contains sympathetics from the intermediolateral cell column, conveyed via the sympathetic chain and parasympathetics from S2–S4 spinal cord levels conveyed via pelvic splanchnics
Prostate		
Overall	Lobes: • Lateral (right and left)—largest, located on sides of prostatic urethra • Isthmus—anterior to urethra, muscular continuation of internal urethral sphincter • Posterior—posterior to urethra, palpable via rectum • Middle—between urethra and ejaculatory ducts; enlargement may interfere with urination	• Surrounds prostatic urethra Possesses fibrous capsule—**fibrous capsule of the prostate,** which invests nerves and vessels supplying the gland and is surrounded by the visceral layer of pelvic fascia—prostatic sheath, puboprostatic ligaments, and the rectovesical septum • Prostatic ducts (20–30) open into **prostatic sinuses** on the side of the **seminal colliculus** in the prostatic urethra where they convey a milky alkaline secretion

(continued)

Internal genitalia of the male *(continued)*

Structure	Description	Significance
Vessels	• Arterial supply: prostatic arteries • Venous drainage is to prostatic plexus associated with the fibrous capsule	• Origin of arteries: internal pudendal, middle rectal, and inferior vesical • Venous plexus drains into internal iliac veins and communicates with internal vertebral and vesical venous plexuses—potential routes for metastasis
Innervation	Innervation is from the pelvic plexus	Contains sympathetics from the intermediolateral cell column, conveyed via the sympathetic chain and parasympathetics from S2–S4 spinal cord levels conveyed via pelvic splanchnics
Bulbourethral Glands (2)		
Overall	Lie posterolateral to the membranous urethra within the external urethral sphincter	The ducts of the bulbourethral glands pierce the perineal membrane to open into the bulbous part of the penile urethra, into which they secrete a mucus-like secretion
Vessels	• Arterial supply: perineal branches • Venous drainage parallels arterial supply	Origin of arteries: internal pudendal
Innervation	Innervation is from the pelvic plexus	Contains sympathetics from the intermediolateral cell column, conveyed via the sympathetic chain and parasympathetics from S2–S4 spinal cord levels conveyed via pelvic splanchnics

Clinical Significance

Vasectomy

The vasectomy (ligation of the ductus deferens) is a common method of sterilization in the male.

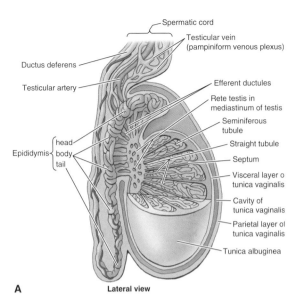

A

Lateral view

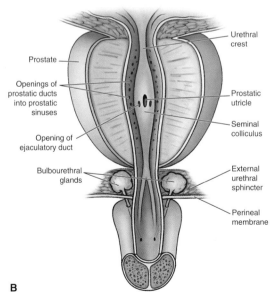

B

FIGURE 3-5. A: Testis and (B) prostate. (From Dudek RW, Louis TM. *High-Yield Gross Anatomy.* 3rd ed. Baltimore: Lippincott Williams & Wilkins; 2008:196.)

Enlargement of the Prostate

Hypertrophy of the prostate is common after middle age and can interfere with urination. The seminal glands and prostate are easily palpable from the rectum. Cancer of the prostate affects 1 in 10 males.

External genitalia of the male
(Figures 3-5 and 3-6)

Structure	Description	Significance
Penile Urethra		
Overall	• Distal to the membranous urethra • Begins at perineal membrane, ends at external urethral orifice • Expansion at proximal end in bulb of penis—the intrabulbar fossa and at distal end—the navicular fossa	• **Membranous urethra** traverses the deep perineal pouch and is surrounded by the **external urethral sphincter** • **Bulbourethral glands** open into proximal part, whereas **urethral glands** open along length to lubricate urethra
Vessels	• Arterial supply: dorsal artery of the penis • Venous supply: parallels arterial supply	Origin of arteries: internal pudendal artery
Innervation	Pudendal nerve	Pain and general tactile impulses conveyed to spinal cord via pudendal nerve
Testes		
Overall	• Located in scrotum • Outer layer—tunica albuginea surrounded by tunica vaginalis • An expansion of tunica albuginea on posterior aspect of testis forms mediastinum testis, which sends septa into testicle to form lobules • Lobules contain seminiferous tubules that join posteriorly as straight tubules that traverse the mediastinum as the rete testis	• Produce sperms and testosterone • **Tunica vaginalis** is an extension of peritoneum, divided into visceral layer on surface of testis and parietal layer lining scrotal wall • Seminiferous tubules are site of sperm production • Leydig cells in interstitial tissue are site of testosterone production • Rete testis convey sperm to head of epididymis via efferent ductules

(continued)

Structure	Description	Significance
Vessels	• Arterial supply: testicular (form part of spermatic cord) • Venous drainage: pampiniform plexus	• Origin of arteries: abdominal aorta • **Pampiniform plexus** helps with temperature regulation for sperm formation and forms the left (empties into left renal vein) and right (empties into inferior vena cava) testicular veins
Innervation	Parasympathetic and sympathetic fibers from testicular plexus	• Parasympathetics: from vagus • Sympathetics: from thoracic spinal cord and paravertebral chain
Penis		
Overall	• Parts: root, body, and glans • Formed of 3 cylinders of erectile tissue: 1 **corpus spongiosum** and 2 **corpora cavernosa** that are surrounded by the **deep fascia of the penis**	• The dorsal corpora cavernosa are surrounded by a thick tunica albuginea that make for rigid erection, they separate into 2 crura proximally and fuse with the ischiopubic rami for support • The ventrally located corpus spongiosum is traversed by the penile urethra and remains less rigid
Vessels	• Arterial supply: deep and dorsal arteries of the penis • Venous drainage: blood from the erectile tissues drains to deep dorsal vein of penis, blood from remaining penile structures drains via the superficial dorsal veins to the external pudendal vein	• Origin of arteries: internal pudendal • Deep dorsal vein conveys blood to the prostatic plexus of veins
Innervation	Receives parasympathetic, sympathetic and sensory fibers	Contain sympathetics from the intermediolateral cell column, conveyed via the sympathetic chain and parasympathetics from S2–S4 spinal cord levels conveyed via pelvic splanchnics, afferents are carried by the dorsal nerve of the penis, a branch of the pudendal nerve

The scrotum is an outpocketing of the anterior abdominal wall and is presented in Chapter 2. The testicles are presented with the male external genitalia.

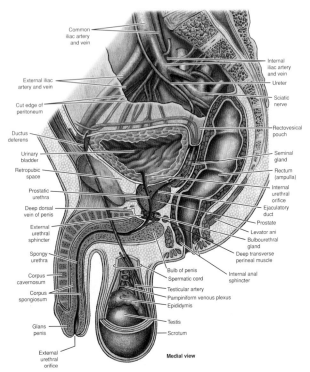

Common
iliac artery
and vein

Internal
iliac artery
and vein

External iliac
artery and vein

Ureter

Cut edge of
peritoneum

Sciatic
nerve

Ductus
deferens

Rectovesical
pouch

Urinary
bladder

Seminal
gland

Retropubic
space

Rectum
(ampulla)

Prostatic
urethra

Internal
urethral
orifice

Deep dorsal
vein of penis

Ejaculatory
duct

External
urethral
sphincter

Prostate

Levator ani

Spongy
urethra

Bulbourethral
gland

Deep transverse
perineal muscle

Corpus
cavernosum

Bulb of penis

Internal anal
sphincter

Corpus
spongiosum

Spermatic cord

Testicular artery

Pampiniform venous plexus

Epididymis

Glans
penis

Testis

Scrotum

External
urethral
orifice

Medial view

FIGURE 3-6. Male midsagittal through pelvis. (From Moore KL, Dalley AF. *Clinically Oriented Anatomy.* 5th ed. Baltimore: Lippincott Williams & Wilkins; 2006:407.)

Additional Concept

Structure of the Penis

The **root** of the penis is located in the superficial pouch and consists of: two crura—each formed of corpora cavernosa, the single bulb—formed of an expanded proximal portion of the corpora spongiosa containing the proximal penile urethra and the muscles covering each—the ischiocavernosus invests the crura, whereas the bulbospongiosus invests the bulb. The **body** (or shaft) of the penis is the main, pendulous part. The body expands on the distal end of the penis to form the **glans** (or head) penis. The glans projects proximally over the corpora to form the **corona**. The skin of the penis extends over the glans forming the **prepuce**. The external urethral orifice opens near the distal tip of the glans.

Penile Support

The penis is supported by the **suspensory ligament of the penis**—an extension of deep fascia that fuses with the deep fascia of the penis. The **fundiform ligament of the penis** is an extension of the membranous layer of superficial fascia, which blends with the superficial fascia of the penis.

Clinical Significance

Erection and Ejaculation

During **erection**, parasympathetic fibers relax the smooth muscles in arteries supplying the corpora cavernosa, allowing blood to flow in, whereas the bulbospongiosus and ischiocavernosus impede venous return. During **ejaculation**, sympathetic fibers close the internal urethral sphincter, parasympathetic fibers cause contraction of the smooth muscle of the urethra and the pudendal nerve causes rhythmic contraction of the bulbospongiosus.

Lymphatic Drainage

The lymphatic drainage of the testes follow the testicular vessels to lumbar lymph nodes, whereas lymphatic drainage of the scrotum is to superficial inguinal lymph nodes.

PERINEUM

Structure of the perineum

Area	Structure	Significance
Overall	Boundaries: • Anterior—pubic symphysis • Posterior—coccyx • Posterolateral—sacrotuberous ligaments • Anterolateral—ischiopubic ramus	• Diamond-shaped area between thighs • Divided into urogenital and anal triangles by a line drawn between the ischial tuberosities

(continued)

Structure of the perineum (continued)

Area	Structure	Significance
Urogenital triangle	Anterior half of the diamond-shaped perineal region	Contains the scrotum and the root of the penis in males and the vulva in females
Anal triangle	Posterior half of the diamond-shaped perineal region	Contains the anal canal and anus and the ischioanal fossae in both sexes
Ischioanal fossae	• Wedge-shaped, fascial spaces between the levator ani (medially), the obturator internus (laterally), and skin of the buttock (inferiorly) • Anterior recess of fossae extend into deep perineal pouch	• The superiorly oriented apex is located along the tendinous arch of the levator ani • Fat-filled space traversed by inferior rectal neurovascular elements • Fat allows for expansion of anal canal, anus and rectum during defecation
Pudendal canal	• Passageway composed of obturator fascia along the lateral wall of the ischioanal fossa • Begins at lesser sciatic notch and ends at the perineal membrane	Conveys pudendal nerve and internal pudendal vessels
Superficial perineal pouch	Space between the perineal membrane and membranous layer of superficial fascia	Contains roots of penis or clitoris, ischiocavernosus and bulbospongiosus, superficial transverse perinei, greater vestibular glands (female), and deep perineal branches of internal pudendal vessels and pudendal nerve
Deep perineal pouch	Space between the perineal membrane and the inferior fascia of the pelvic diaphragm	Contains anterior recess of ischioanal fossa, deep transverse perinei, external urethral sphincter, and part of the urethra (and bulbourethral glands in the male)

The rectum and anal canal are presented with the large intestine in Chapter 2.

Additional Concept

Pudendal Neurovascular Elements

Before entering the **pudendal canal**, the **pudendal nerve** and **internal pudendal vessels** give off **inferior rectal** branches that course across the fossa to the rectum, anal canal, and anus. The pudendal nerve and internal pudendal vessels terminate by dividing into **perineal** (superficial pouch structures), **dorsal artery and nerve of the penis or clitoris** branches (deep pouch structures), and **posterior scrotal or labial branches.**

Fascia of the perineum

Fascia/Connective Tissue	Significance/Structure
Membranous layer of superficial fascia (Colles')	• Along the posterior edge of the urogenital membrane, fuses with the perineal membrane and perineal body • Laterally, fuses with the fascia lata of the thigh; anteriorly, it is continuous with the membranous layer of superficial fascia of the abdomen (Scarpa's)
Perineal membrane	• Deep fascia spanning the urogenital triangle, investing the bulbospongiosus, ischiocavernosus, and transverse perinei muscles • Pierced by the urethra and the vagina in the female • Forms roof of **superficial perineal pouch**
Perineal body	• Fibromuscular mass between the anus and perineal membrane • Serves as an attachment for bulbospongiosus, transverse perineal muscles, external anal sphincter, and levator ani

Additional Concept

The fatty layer of superficial fascia in the perineum is continuous with the fatty layer over the abdomen and makes up the bulk of the two **labia majora** and **mons pubis** in females.

Clinical Significance

Episiotomy

Damage to the perineal body as may occur during childbirth, trauma, disease, or infection may lead to prolapse of the pelvic viscera. An episiotomy is performed during childbirth to enlarge the vaginal orifice and spare lasting damage to the perineal body.

Muscles of the perineum

Muscle	Proximal Attachment	Distal Attachment	Innervation	Main Actions
Bulbo-spongiosus	Male—perineal body and median raphe; female—perineal body	Male—perineal membrane, corpora spongiosum, and cavernosa and fascia of bulb of penis; female—fascia of bulbs of vestibule	Deep perineal	Male—assists in erection and ejaculation and emptying of urethra after micturition; female—assists in erection
Ischiocav-ernosus	Ischiopubic rami and ischial tuberosities	Crura of penis or clitoris		Maintains erection of penis or clitoris
External anal sphincter	Coccyx via anococcygeal ligament and skin around anus	Perineal body, surrounds anus	Inferior rectal	Closes anus, supports perineal body and pelvic floor
External urethral sphincter	Ischiopubic rami and ischial tuberosities	Surrounds urethra; males—ascends to prostate, females—forms utero-vaginal sphincter	Deep perineal	Compresses urethra for the maintenance of urinary continence
Deep transverse perineal		Perineal body		Fixes perineal body to support pelvic viscera and resist intra-abdominal pressure
Superficial transverse perineal	Ischial tuberosities			

▮ INTRODUCTION

The back consists of the vertebral column, spinal cord and nerves, and the muscles responsible for posture and movement of the vertebral column.

VERTEBRAL COLUMN

Vertebral column structure

The vertebral column is composed of intervertebral disks and 33 vertebrae:

- 7 cervical
- 12 thoracic
- 5 lumbar
- 5 fused sacral
- 4 fused coccygeal

The vertebral column protects the spinal cord and spinal nerves and supports the weight of the body.

Curvatures of the vertebral column

Curvature	Description	Significance
Cervical	• Concave posteriorly (lordosis)	Provide resiliency to vertebral column
Lumbar	• Secondary curvatures—cervical develops when infant begins to hold up head, lumbar develops when infant begins to walk	
Thoracic	• Concave anteriorly (kyphosis)	
Sacral	• Primary curvatures—present at birth	

Additional Concept

Axial and Appendicular Skeleton

The **axial skeleton** is composed of the vertebral column, cranium, and thoracic cage (ribs, sternum, and hyoid bone). The **appendicular skeleton** is everything else (pectoral and pelvic girdles and the limbs).

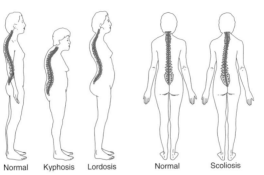

Normal   Kyphosis   Lordosis   Normal   Scoliosis

FIGURE 4-1. Curvatures of the vertebral column. (From Dudek RW, Louis TM. *High-Yield Gross Anatomy.* 3rd ed. Baltimore: Lippincott Williams & Wilkins; 2008:2.)

Clinical Significance

Excess Curvature

Excess thoracic kyphosis (humpback) is often caused by osteoporosis. Excess lumbar lordosis (sway back) is often seen in pregnancy. Scoliosis (crooked back) is a common lateral deformity of the vertebral column in pubertal girls.

Structure of the vertebrae

The vertebrae generally increase in size as progress inferiorly, a reflection of the increasing weight of the body. Vertebrae possess regional characteristics.

Vertebrae	Characteristic	Significance
Typical	Body	• Most anterior; supports body weight, progressively larger as move inferiorly down column • Covered on superior and inferior surface by hyaline cartilage • Peripheral border possesses **epiphysial rim**—a slight elevation that provide attachment for the annuli fibrosi of the intervertebral discs
	Vertebral arch	• Posterior to the body • Formed by a pair of lamina and a pair of pedicles • With the posterior aspect of the body, forms the **vertebral foramen**—contains spinal cord

(continued)

Structure of the vertebrae *(continued)*

Vertebrae	Characteristic	Significance
	Lamina	• Pair of platelike processes that form the posterior part of vertebral arch • Meet posteriorly in the midline
	Pedicle	• Pair of short processes that join vertebral arch to body • Form anterior part of vertebral arch • Notch on superior and inferior surfaces—**vertebral notches:** successive vertebral notches form **intervertebral foramina,** which permit passage of nerve roots and vessels
	Spinous process	• Midline posterior projection from junction of laminae • Allows for muscle and ligament attachments
	Transverse processes (2)	• Project posterolaterally from vertebral arch • Allow for muscle attachment and articulation with ribs (thoracic)
	Superior articular processes (2)	• Arise from junction of pedicles and laminae • Possess facet (zygapophysial) joints for articulation with adjacent processes • Limit undo movement of vertebral column and maintain vertebral alignment
	Inferior articular processes (2)	
Identifying Regional Characteristics		
Cervical	Body	Superior surfaces possess **uncinate process**
	Spinous process	• Bifid • C7, long—**vertebra prominens**
	Transverse process	Possess transverse foramina for passage of vertebral vessels and sympathetic fibers
Thoracic	Spinous process	Long, inferiorly directed
	Transverse process	Possess facets for articulation with head and tubercle of ribs
Lumbar	Body	Massive for weight bearing
	Spinous process	Short and stout
Sacral	Fused	• 5 sacral vertebrae fuse to form sacrum • Remnants of characteristics typical to vertebrae are still identifiable
Coccygeal	Fused	Remnant of taillike caudal eminence

Additional Concept

Vertebral (Spinal) Canal

Adjacent **vertebral foramina** form the **vertebral canal**—contain the spinal cord, meninges, nerve roots, vascular elements (internal venous plexus), and fat.

Clinical Concept

Spina Bifida

Failure of the **vertebral arches** to form correctly results in **spina bifida**; spina bifida occulta (a mild form) is often asymptomatic. More serious forms may result in herniation of meninges—meningocele or meninges and neural tissue through the deficiency.

Vertebral Artery

The long, tortuous course of the vertebral artery through the transverse cervical foramina may increase risk of insult because of stretch from rotation of the head, resulting in reduced blood flow to the brain, possibly causing dizziness and light-headedness.

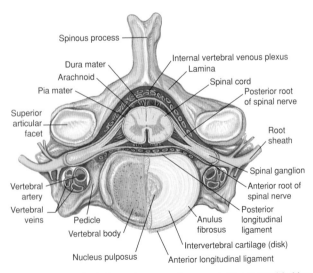

FIGURE 4-2. Typical vertebra, superior aspect. (Asset provided by Anatomical Chart Company.)

Joints of the back
(Figure 4-2)

Joint	Type	Articulation	Structure
Atlanto-occipital	Synovial	C1 vertebra with occipital bone	• Strengthened by **anterior** and **posterior atlanto-occipital membranes**
Atlantoaxial— 2 lateral and 1 median	Lateral— synovial; median— pivot	C1 with C2 vertebrae	• Strengthened and maintained by the **cruciform ligament**— formed by **longitudinal bands** and the **transverse ligament of the atlas** • **Alar ligaments**—prevent excessive rotation • The **tectorial membrane**— continuation of posterior longitudinal ligament, covers the alar and transverse ligaments
Intervertebral	Cartilaginous	Surfaces of adjacent vertebrae connected by intervertebral discs	• **Intervertebral discs** provide strong attachment between adjacent vertebral bodies— consist of outer fibrocartilaginous **anulus fibrosis** (attaches to epiphysial rim) and central compressible **nucleus pulposus** • **Anterior** and **posterior longitudinal ligaments** strengthen, provide stability, and limit extension and flexion of the vertebral column, respectively
Uncovertebral	Synovial	Adjacent cervical vertebrae	Uncinate process on superior surface of cervical vertebral bodies with inferior surface of vertebral body superior to it
Zygapophysial (facet)		Between superior and inferior articulating processes of adjacent vertebrae	• Strengthened by accessory ligaments • Allow for gliding movements

Additional Concept

Multiple accessory ligaments help to strengthen and support the joints of the vertebral column:

- **ligamentum flavum**—connects adjacent vertebral arches
- **supraspinous**—connects adjacent spinous processes
- **interspinous**—connects adjacent spinous processes
- **ligamentum nuchae**—connects external occipital protuberance and cervical spinous processes
- **intertransverse ligaments**—connects adjacent transverse processes

Clinical Significance

Slipped Disc

Herniation of the nucleus pulposus into or through the anulus fibrosis is a common cause of lower back pain and is often called a **slipped** or **ruptured disk.**

SPINAL CORD

Structure of the spinal cord
(Figure 4-2)

The spinal cord is continuous superiorly with the medulla at the foramen magnum and ends inferiorly at the L1–L2 vertebral level. The spinal cord serves as a reflex center and conduction pathway, connecting the brain to the periphery. It is located within the vertebral canal and gives rise to 31 pairs of spinal nerves.

Feature	Description	Significance
Cervical enlargement	Enlarged portion of spinal cord from C4–T1	Gives rise to the anterior rami that form the **brachial plexus**—innervates upper limbs
Lumbar enlargement	Enlarged portion of spinal cord from L1–S3	Gives rise to the anterior rami that form the **lumbosacral plexus**—innervates lower limbs
Medullary cone	Tapering end of the spinal cord	• Located at L1–L2 vertebral level • Nerve roots contribute to cauda equina
Cauda equina	Formed from anterior and posterior roots that arise from the lumbar enlargement and medullary cone	Located in the **lumbar cistern**—continuation of subarachnoid space in the **dural sac** caudal to the medullary cone
Spinal nerves (31 pairs)	• 8 cervical, 12 thoracic, 5 lumbar, 5 sacral, 1 coccygeal	• Formed of anterior and posterior roots from the spinal cord segments

(continued)

Structure of the spinal cord *(continued)*

Feature	Description	Significance
	• Each contains somatic afferent and efferent fibers and between T1–L2 contain presynaptic sympathetic fibers, between S2–S4 contain presynaptic parasympathetic fibers	• Terminate by dividing into anterior and posterior primary rami
Roots—anterior and posterior	• Anterior—efferent • Posterior—afferent • Join to form spinal nerves	• Anterior roots contain fibers of somatic and visceral motor neurons • Posterior roots contain somatic and visceral afferent fibers
Spinal ganglion	Located along posterior root	Contains primary afferent cell bodies of the somatic and visceral sensory systems
Gray matter	Located on the inside of the spinal cord, deep to the white matter	Divided into posterior, lateral (visceral motor, between T1–L2), and anterior (somatic motor) horns
White matter	Located on the outside of the spinal cord, superficial to the gray matter	• Divided into anterior, lateral, and posterior funiculi • Contains ascending (afferent) and descending (efferent) fiber tracts
Rami—anterior and posterior	Terminal branches of spinal nerves	• Anterior—supply innervation to majority of body, often form plexuses • Posterior—supply segmental innervation to the back

Vessels of the spinal cord
(Figure 4-2)

Artery	Origin	Description
Anterior spinal	Vertebral	Supplies anterior 2/3 of spinal cord superiorly
Posterior spinal (2)	Either vertebral or posterior inferior cerebellar	Supplies posterior 1/3 of spinal cord superiorly
Segmental	Ascending cervical, deep cervical, vertebral, posterior intercostal and lumbar	• Enter vertebral canal through intervertebral foramina • Supply spinal cord and coverings segmentally • Anastomose with spinal arteries

(continued)

Vessels of the spinal cord *(continued)*

Artery	Origin	Description
Radicular—anterior and posterior	Segmental	Supply nerve roots and associated meninges
Medullary		• Variable, but prevalent in the region of the cervical and lumbosacral enlargements • Supplement spinal arterial supply

Vein	Termination	Description
Anterior spinal (3)	Drained by medullary and radicular veins	• Generally parallel arterial supply • Eventually drain into the internal vertebral venous plexus
Posterior spinal (3)		
Medullary	Drain into internal vertebral venous plexus	
Radicular		
Internal vertebral venous plexus	Drain into dural sinuses of cranial vault	• Communicates with external venous plexus on external aspect of vertebrae • Potential route for infection spread from cranial vault

Structure of spinal cord meninges
(Figure 4-2)

The spinal cord meninges support and protect the nerve roots and form the subarachnoid space. From superficial to deep:

- dura mater
- arachnoid mater
- pia mater

Structure	Description	Significance
Dura mater	• Outer layer of meninges • Continuous with meningeal layer of cranial dura superiorly	• Tough, fibrous layer • Separated from vertebrae by epidural space
Epidural space	Between vertebrae and dura mater	Contains fat and the internal vertebral venous plexus
Dural root sheaths	Extensions of the dural sac that cover spinal nerve roots and spinal nerves	• Sheaths end by blending with the epineurium of the spinal nerves • Extend through intervertebral foramina

(continued)

Structure of spinal cord meninges *(continued)*

Structure	Description	Significance
Dural sac	Long tubular sac that contains the spinal cord and cerebrospinal fluid	Begins at the **foramen magnum,** anchored to coccyx by filum terminale
Subdural space	• Potential space, between the dura and arachnoid mater • Filled with a loosely adhered cell layer	Site of subdural hematoma when trauma causes bleeding into space
Arachnoid mater	• Middle meningeal layer • Encloses the subarachnoid space	Lines dural sac and dural root sheaths
Subarachnoid space	Between arachnoid mater and pia mater	• Contains cerebrospinal fluid, arachnoid trabeculae, and blood vessels • Inferior prolongation forms the lumbar cistern
Arachnoid trabeculae	Connective tissue strands that connect the arachnoid and pia mater	Span the subarachnoid space
Lumbar cistern	Inferior prolongation of the subarachnoid space	Contains the **cauda equina** and **filum terminale** internus
Pia mater	• Delicate inner (deep) meninge in contact with the spinal cord • Deep to the subarachnoid space	Invests spinal blood vessels and the roots of the spinal nerves
Denticulate ligaments	• 21 pairs • Lateral extensions of pia mater between the anterior and posterior roots	Anchors spinal cord to the dura mater
Filum terminale—internus and externus	• Inferior extension of pia mater • Extends from medullary cone to inferior aspect of dural sac (interna) and to the tip of the coccyx (externa)	Anchors inferior end of spinal cord to dura mater and coccyx

Clinical Significance

Anesthesia

Epidural anesthesia entails injection of a local anesthetic around the sacral spinal nerves, external to the dural sac.

Spinal Tap and Block

A **lumbar puncture** (spinal tap) is performed for extraction of cerebrospinal fluid from the lumbar cistern for examination. A **spinal block** entails introduction of an anesthetic into the cerebrospinal fluid through a lumbar puncture.

MUSCULATURE

Muscles of the back

The muscles located on the back are divided into extrinsic and intrinsic. The **extrinsic muscles** of the back are discussed with the upper limb (superficial layer) and thorax (intermediate layer), with which they are associated functionally.

Intrinsic Back Muscle	Proximal Attachment	Distal Attachment	Innervation	Main Actions
Superficial Layer				
Splenius—capitis and cervicis	Nuchal ligament and C7–T4 vertebrae	• Capitis—mastoid process and superior nuchal line • Cervicis—transverse processes of C1–C4 vertebrae	Segmental innervation by posterior rami of spinal nerves	• Laterally flex neck and rotate head • Extend head and neck when contracting bilaterally
Intermediate Layer (Erector Spinae)				
Iliocostalis—lumborum, thoracis, and cervicis	Arise as fused muscle mass from iliac crest and sacrum, sacroiliac ligaments, and spinous processes of sacral and lumbar vertebrae	Angles of lower ribs and transverse processes of thoracic and cervical vertebrae	Segmental innervation by posterior rami of spinal nerves	Laterally flex vertebral column; extend vertebral column (chief extensor of column) and head, control flexion by gradual relaxation of fibers when acting bilaterally
Longissimus—thoracis, cervicis and capitis		Angles of ribs and transverse processes of thoracic and		

(continued)

Muscles of the back (continued)

Intrinsic Back Muscle	Proximal Attachment	Distal Attachment	Innervation	Main Actions
		cervical vertebrae and mastoid process		
Spinalis—thoracis, cervicis, and capitis		Spinous processes of upper thoracic vertebrae and cranium		
Deep Layer (Transversospinal Group)				
Semispinalis—thoracis, cervicis and capitis	Transverse processes C4–T12	Spinous processes of 4–6 vertebrae superior and occipital bone	Segmental innervation by posterior rami of spinal nerves	• Extends thoracic and cervical regions of vertebral column and head • Rotates vertebral column
Multifidus	Posterior sacrum, posterior iliac spine, transverse processes T1–T3 and articular processes of C4–C7	Spinous processes of 2–4 vertebrae superior		Stabilizes vertebrae
Rotators—brevis and longus	Transverse processes	Junction of lamina and transverse process or spinous processes of 1 (brevis), 2 (longus) vertebrae superior		
Interspinales	Spinous processes	Spinous processes of		Extension and rotation of

(continued)

Muscles of the back *(continued)*

Intrinsic Back Muscle	Proximal Attachment	Distal Attachment	Innervation	Main Actions
	of cervical and lumbar vertebrae	vertebrae immediately superior		vertebral column
Intertrans-versarii	Transverse processes of cervical and lumbar vertebrae	Transverse processes of adjacent vertebrae		Lateral flexion and stabilization of vertebral column
Levator costarum	Transverse processes of C7–T11 vertebrae	Adjacent rib between tubercle and angle		Elevate ribs, assist in lateral flexion of vertebral column

Additional Concept

The muscles of the back may be divided into 3 layers: superficial—associated with the upper limb; intermediate—associated with the thorax; and deep—associated with movement of the vertebral column. They are also known as the **intrinsic muscles of the back** or true back muscles.

Mnemonic

Erector Spinae Muscles

From lateral to medial:

I Like Spaghetti
Iliocostalis
Longissimus
Spinalis

Suboccipital triangle

The suboccipital triangle is a muscular triangle inferior to the occipital region of the head; it contains the vertebral artery, posterior arch of the atlas, and the suboccipital nerve (C1).

Suboccipital Region	Structure	Significance
Borders	• Roof—semispinalis capitis • Floor—atlanto-occipital membrane and arch of C1	• Identifiable muscular triangle in the

(continued)

Suboccipital triangle *(continued)*

Suboccipital Region	Structure	Significance
	• Superomedial—rectus capitis posterior major • Superolateral—superior oblique • Inferolateral—inferior oblique	suboccipital region
Muscles		
Rectus capitis posterior major	• Proximal attachment: C2 spinous process • Distal attachment: inferior nuchal line of occipital bone	• Actions: extend and rotate head • Innervation: suboccipital nerve (C1)
Rectus capitis posterior minor	• Proximal attachment: C1 posterior arch • Distal attachment: inferior nuchal line of occipital bone	
Inferior oblique of the head	• Proximal attachment: C2 spinous process • Distal attachment: C1 transverse process	
Superior oblique of the head	• Proximal attachment: C1 transverse process • Distal attachment: occipital bone	

5

Lower Limb

The pelvic (anterior) aspect of the bones of the gluteal region are described in Chapters 3 and 4.

■ INTRODUCTION

The lower limb is divided for descriptive purposes by skeletal elements into:

- gluteal region—portion between thigh and trunk posteriorly that includes the pelvic girdle: ilium, ischium, and pubis
- thigh—portion between the gluteal region posteriorly and the knee that includes the femur
- leg—portion between the knee and ankle that includes the tibia and fibula
- foot—portion distal to the ankle that includes the metatarsals and phalanges; the tarsal bones form the ankle

GLUTEAL REGION

Bones of the gluteal region
(Figure 5-1)

Bone	Feature	Significance
Sacrum	Median crest	Fused spinal processes of sacral vertebrae
	Posterior sacral foramina	Transmit posterior rami of first 4 sacral nerves
	Sacral hiatus	Inferior opening of the vertebral canal between the sacral cornu (horns)
Coccyx	Apex of the coccyx	• Directed inferiorly • Coccyx is formed by the fusion of the 4 inferiormost vertebrae
Hip Bone (Pelvic Bone, Coxal Bone)—Fusion of the 3 Bones Below		
Ilium	Body of ilium	Contributes to the acetabulum
	Wing (ala) of ilium	• Concave surface • Marked by the anterior, posterior, and inferior gluteal lines

(continued)

Bones of the gluteal region (continued)

Bone	Characteristic	Significance
	Iliac crest	• Bony ridge between the anterior superior, and posterior superior iliac spines • Attachment for fascia lata, tensor of fascia lata, external oblique, internal oblique, transverse abdominal, latissimus dorsi, quadratus lumborum, erector spinae, and iliacus
	Posterior superior iliac spine	Attachment for sacroiliac ligaments and multifidus
	Posterior inferior iliac spine	Part of auricular surface of ilium
	Anterior gluteal line	• Gluteus medius attaches between anterior and posterior gluteal lines • Gluteus minimus attaches between anterior and inferior gluteal lines
	Posterior gluteal line	• Gluteus maximus attaches posterior to the posterior gluteal line • Gluteus medius attaches between anterior and posterior gluteal lines
	Inferior gluteal line	Gluteus minimus attaches between anterior and inferior gluteal lines
	Greater sciatic notch/foramen	• Notch converted into greater sciatic foramen by the sacrospinous ligament • Major passageway for structures exiting the pelvis and entering the gluteal region—including: piriformis, superior and inferior gluteal vessels and nerves, sciatic and posterior femoral cutaneous nerves, internal pudendal vessels, pudendal nerve and nerves to obturator internus, and quadratus femoris
Ischium	Ischial spine	Attachment for superior gemellus and sacrospinous ligament
	Ischial tuberosity	Attachment for hamstring portion of adductor magnus, hamstrings, and sacrotuberous ligament
	Body	Contributes to the acetabulum
	Lesser sciatic notch/foramen	• Notch converted into lesser sciatic foramen by the sacrospinous and sacrotuberous ligaments • Passageway for structures exiting and entering the perineum—tendon of obturator internus (exiting), internal pudendal vessels, and pudendal nerve (entering)
Pubis	Body	Contributes to the acetabulum

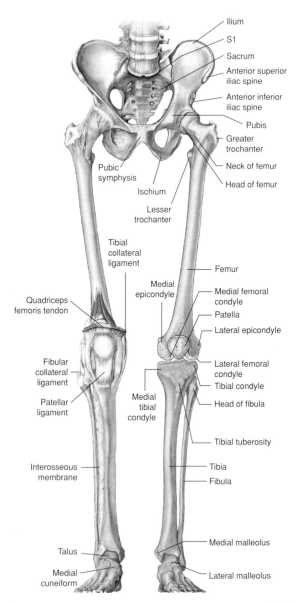

FIGURE 5-1. Lower limb bones. Anterior view. (Asset provided by Anatomical Chart Company.)

Additional Concept

Acetabulum

The **acetabulum** is formed by the bodies of the pubis, ischium, and ilium; it forms the socket of the hip joint.

Clinical Significance

Contusion of the iliac crest is known as a "hip pointer."

Muscles of the gluteal region

Muscle	Proximal Attachment	Distal Attachment	Innervation	Main Actions
Gluteus maximus	Ilium posterior to posterior gluteal line, sacrum, coccyx; and sacrotuberous ligament	Iliotibial tract and gluteal tuberosity	Inferior gluteal	• Extends and laterally rotates thigh • Steadies thigh
Gluteus medius	Ilium between anterior and posterior gluteal lines	Greater trochanter of femur	Superior gluteal	• Abducts and medially rotates thigh • Levels pelvis when contralateral leg is unsupported
Gluteus minimus	Ilium between anterior and inferior gluteal lines			
Tensor of fascia lata	Anterior superior iliac spine	Lateral condyle of tibia via iliotibial tract		
Piriformis	Sacrum and sacrotuberous ligament	Greater trochanter of femur	Sacral plexus (S1 and S2)	• Laterally rotates thigh • Assist in holding head of femur in acetabulum
Obturator internus	Margins of obturator foramen and obturator membrane		Nerve to obturator internus	
Superior gemellus	Ischial spine			
Inferior gemellus	Ischial tuberosity		Nerve to quadratus femoris	
Quadratus femoris		Intertrochanteric crest		

Clinical Significance

The gluteal region is a common site for intramuscular injection; injections are made in the superolateral quadrant to avoid neurovascular elements.

Mnemonic
Lateral Rotators of the Hip Joint

Play Golf Or Go On Quaaludes
Piriformis
Gemellus superior
Obturator internus
Gemellus inferior
Obturator externus
Quadratus femoris

Nerves of the gluteal region

Nerve	Origin	Structures Innervated
Superior gluteal	Sacral plexus	Gluteus medius, gluteus minimus, tensor of fascia lata
Inferior gluteal		Gluteus maximus
Pudendal		Supplies the perineum; supplies no structures in the gluteal region
Sciatic		Supplies the lower limb; supplies no structures in the gluteal region
Nerve to quadratus femoris		Quadratus femoris and inferior gemellus
Nerve to obturator internus		Obturator internus and superior gemellus
Posterior femoral cutaneous		Skin of gluteal region
Superior clunial	L1–L3	
Middle clunial	S1–S3	
Inferior clunial	S2–S3	
Iliohypogastric	Lumbar plexus	Skin of buttock

Vessels of the gluteal region
(Figure 5-2)

Artery	Origin	Description
Superior gluteal	Internal iliac	Supplies gluteus maximus, gluteus medius, gluteus minimus, and tensor of fascia lata
Inferior gluteal		• Supplies gluteus maximus, obturator internus, and quadratus femoris • Participates in cruciate anastomosis with the deep femoral (1st perforating branch) and the medial and lateral circumflex arteries
Internal pudendal		• Supplies structures in the perineal region • Supplies no structures in the gluteal region

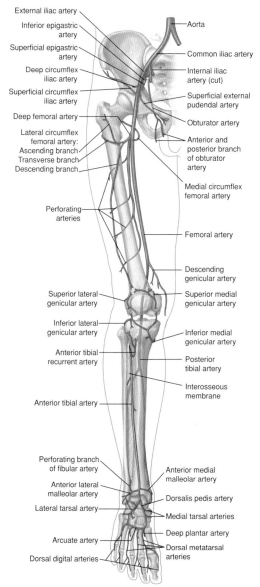

FIGURE 5-2. Arteries of lower limb, anterior view. (From Tank PW, Gest TR. *LWW Atlas of Anatomy.* Baltimore: Lippincott Williams & Wilkins; 2009:148.)

Additional Concept

Venous Drainage

The venous drainage generally parallels arterial supply.

THIGH REGION

Bones of the thigh
(Figures 5-1 and 5-2)

Bone	Feature	Significance
Femur (thigh bone)	Head	• Articulates with acetabulum • Bears a fovea for attachment of the ligament of the head of the femur
	Neck	Attachment for the capsule of the hip joint
	Greater trochanter	Attachment for gluteus medius and minimus, piriformis, obturator internus, superior and inferior gemelli, and vastus lateralis
	Lesser trochanter	Attachment for iliacus and psoas major
	Trochanteric fossa	Attachment for obturator externus
	Intertrochanteric line	Attachment for iliofemoral ligament and vastus medialis
	Intertrochanteric crest	Attachment for quadratus femoris
	Linea aspera	Attachment for pectineus, iliacus, vastus medialis and lateralis, adductor magnus, longus and brevis, biceps femoris (short head), and gluteus maximus
	Gluteal tuberosity	Attachment for gluteus maximus
	Adductor tubercle	• Associated with the medial epicondyle • Attachment for adductor magnus
	Shaft	Attachment for vastus intermedius
	Medial condyle	Articulate with tibial plateau
	Lateral condyle	
	Intercondylar fossa	• Depression between medial and lateral condyles • Attachment for anterior and posterior cruciate ligaments
	Medial epicondyle	• Attachment for tibial collateral ligament, gastrocnemius • Bears adductor tubercle
	Lateral epicondyle	Attachment for fibular collateral ligament, gastrocnemius, plantaris, and popliteus

Clinical Significance

Coxa Vara and Coxa Valga

When the angle of inclination between the neck and shaft of the femur is decreased, the condition is coxa vara; when it is increased, it is coxa valga.

Femoral Fracture

Femoral fractures often occur at the neck; spiral fractures occur in the shaft of the femur.

Muscles of the thigh

Muscle	Proximal Attachment	Distal Attachment	Innervation	Main Actions
Anterior Compartment—Hip Flexors and Knee Extensors				
Pectineus	Pubis	Pectineal line of femur	Femoral or obturator	Adducts, flexes, and medially rotates thigh
Psoas major	T12 and lumbar vertebrae	Lesser trochanter of femur	Segmental (L1–L3)	Flexes thigh and stabilizes hip joint
Psoas minor	T12–L1	Pectineal line	Segmental	
Iliacus	Iliac fossa	Lesser trochanter of femur	Femoral	
Sartorius	Anterior superior iliac spine	Medial condyle of tibia via **pes anserinus**		Flexes, abducts and laterally rotates thigh, flexes leg
Rectus femoris	Anterior inferior iliac spine	Tibial tuberosity via patellar ligament		Extends leg, flexes thigh, and stabilizes hip joint
Vastus lateralis	Greater trochanter and linea aspera of femur			Extends leg
Vastus medialis	Intertrochanteric line and linea aspera of femur			
Vastus intermedius	Femoral shaft			

(continued)

Muscles of the thigh *(continued)*

Muscle	Proximal Attachment	Distal Attachment	Innervation	Main Actions
Medial Compartment—Thigh Adductors				
Adductor longus	Pubis	Linea aspera of femur	Obturator	Adducts thigh
Adductor brevis				
Adductor magnus	• Adductor portion: pubis • Hamstring portion: ischial tuberosity	• Adductor portion: gluteal tuberosity and linea aspera • Hamstring portion: adductor tubercle of femur	• Adductor portion: obturator • Hamstring portion: tibial division of sciatic	• Adductor portion: adducts thigh • Hamstring portion: extends thigh
Gracilis	Pubis	Medial condyle of tibia via *pes anserinus*	Obturator	Adducts thigh, flexes and medially rotates leg
Obturator externus	Margins of obturator foramen and obturator membrane—externally	Trochanteric fossa of femur		• Laterally rotates thigh • Holds head of femur in acetabulum
Posterior Compartment—Knee Flexors and Hip Extensors				
Semitendinosus	Ischial tuberosity	Medial condyle of tibia via *pes anserinus*	Tibial division of sciatic	Extend thigh, flex and medially rotate leg
Semimembranosus		Medial condyle of tibia		
Biceps femoris	• Long head: ischial tuberosity • Short head: linea aspera	Head of fibula	• Long head: tibial division of sciatic • Short head: common fibular division of sciatic	Flexes and laterally rotates leg, flexes thigh

Additional Concept

Quadriceps Femoris

The rectus femoris, vastus lateralis, vastus medialis, and vastus intermedius are collectively referred to as the **quadriceps femoris**.

Hamstrings

The semitendinosus, semimembranosus, and biceps femoris are collectively referred to as the **hamstrings**.

Clinical Significance

Cramp

A cramp or spasm in the anterior thigh muscles—a "Charley Horse"—usually involves the rectus femoris.

Gracilis

Gracilis is sometimes transplanted to replace damaged muscles elsewhere in the body.

Groin pull

A groin pull usually refers to straining the proximal aspect of the musculature of the medial compartment of the thigh.

Mnemonics

Adductor Magnus

AM SO: Adductor Magnus innervated by Sciatic and Obturator.

Pes Anserinus

Pes Anserinus—Say Grace before Serving Tea

Sartorius
Gracilis
Semitendinosus

Nerves of the thigh

Nerve	Origin	Structures Innervated
Femoral	Lumbar plexus	• Pectineus, sartorius, iliacus, rectus femoris, vastus lateralis, medialis, and intermedius • Sensory to skin over anteromedial thigh
Obturator		Adductor longus, adductor brevis, gracilis, pectineus, obturator externus, and adductor magnus

(continued)

Nerves of the thigh *(continued)*

Nerve	Origin	Structures Innervated
Tibial division of sciatic	Sciatic	Long head of biceps femoris, semitendinosus, semimembranosus
Common fibular division of sciatic		Short head of biceps femoris
Genitofemoral	Lumbar plexus	Sensory to skin of inguinal region
Lateral femoral cutaneous		Sensory to skin over lateral thigh
Posterior femoral cutaneous	Sacral plexus	Sensory to skin of gluteal region and posterior thigh

Vessels of the thigh
(Figure 5-2)

Artery	Origin	Description
Internal pudendal	Internal iliac	Supplies external genitals and perineal region
Obturator		• Divides into anterior and posterior branches • The posterior branch gives rise to the acetabular branch and the artery to the head of the femur • Both branches supply the adductor compartment of the thigh
Femoral	Continuation of external iliac	• Gives rise to deep femoral, superficial epigastric, superficial circumflex iliac, external pudendal, medial and lateral femoral circumflex, and descending genicular • Terminates by becoming the popliteal artery after passing through the adductor hiatus
Deep femoral	Femoral	• Gives rise to 4 perforating branches that supply adductor magnus and hamstrings • 1st perforating branch participates in cruciate anastomosis with the inferior gluteal and the medial and lateral circumflex arteries
Superficial epigastric		Supplies subcutaneous tissues—lymph nodes, skin, and fascia over the abdominal wall
Superficial circumflex iliac		Supplies subcutaneous tissues—lymph nodes, skin, and fascia over the inguinal region

(continued)

Vessels of the thigh (continued)

Artery	Origin	Description
Superficial external pudendal		Supplies subcutaneous tissues—skin and fascia over the external genitals
Deep external pudendal		
Medial femoral circumflex	Deep femoral	• Supplies most of the blood to the head and neck of femur • Participates in cruciate anastomosis with the inferior gluteal, lateral circumflex, and 1st perforating branch of the deep femoral
Lateral femoral circumflex		• Supplies neck of femur and contributes to anastomosis around knee joint • Participates in cruciate anastomosis with the inferior gluteal, medial circumflex, and 1st perforating branch of the deep femoral
Descending genicular	Femoral	Supplies subcutaneous tissue on medial aspect of knee and contributes to anastomosis around knee

Additional Concept
Venous Drainage
Venous drainage generally follows arterial supply.

Clinical Significance
Femoral Artery
The proximal portion of the femoral artery is easily accessible and easily damaged because of its superficial location.

LEG REGION

Leg bones
(Figures 5-1, 5-4, and 5-5)

Bone	Feature	Significance
Tibia	Medial condyle	• Articulates with femoral condyles • Attachment for semimembranosus and tibial collateral ligament

(continued)

Leg bones (continued)

Bone	Feature	Significance
	Lateral condyle	• Articulates with femoral condyles • Attachment for iliotibial band
	Anterior intercondylar area	• Located between the condyles • Provide attachment sites for anterior and posterior cruciate ligaments and the menisci
	Posterior intercondylar area	
	Tuberosity of the tibia	Attachment for patellar ligament
	Shaft	Attachment for tibial collateral ligament, popliteus, soleus, flexor digitorum longus, interosseous membrane, gracilis, and semitendinosus
	Soleal line	Attachment for popliteus, soleus, flexor digitorum longus, and tibialis posterior
	Medial malleolus	• Attachment for deltoid ligament • Lateral surface articulates with the talus
Fibula	Head	Attachment for biceps femoris, fibular collateral ligament, fibularis longus, extensor digitorum longus, and soleus
	Neck	Common fibular nerve wraps around neck to access the anterior aspect of the leg
	Shaft	Attachment for interosseous membrane, extensor digitorum longus, extensor hallucis longus, soleus, tibialis posterior, fibularis longus, brevis, and tertius
	Lateral malleolus	• Medial surface articulates with the talus • Attachment for the posterior and anterior talofibular ligaments and the calcaneofibular ligament

Clinical Significance

Fractures

Tibia

The most common site for a fracture of the **tibia** is along the shaft at the junction of its middle and inferior thirds; it is the narrowest part and has a relatively poor blood supply.

Fibula

Fracture of the **fibula** often occurs proximal to the lateral malleolus and is often associated with fracture dislocations of the ankle joint.

Muscles of the leg

Muscle	Proximal Attachment	Distal Attachment	Innervation	Main Actions
Anterior Compartment				
Tibialis anterior	Tibia and interosseous membrane	1st metatarsal	Deep fibular	Dorsiflexes ankle, inverts foot
Extensor digitorum longus		Middle and distal phalanges digits 2–5		Extends digits 2–5, dorsiflexes ankle
Extensor hallucis longus	Fibula and interosseous membrane	Distal phalanx digit 1		Extends digit 1, dorsiflexes ankle
Fibularis tertius		5th metatarsal		Dorsiflexes ankle, everts foot
Lateral Compartment				
Fibularis longus	Fibula	1st metatarsal	Superficial fibular	Plantarflex ankle, evert foot
Fibularis brevis		Tuberosity of 5th metatarsal		
Posterior Compartment				
Gastrocnemius	Femoral condyles	Calcaneus via calcaneal tendon	Tibial	Flexes leg, plantarflexes ankle
Soleus	Soleal line of tibia and fibula			Plantarflexes ankle
Plantaris	Oblique popliteal ligament and lateral supracondylar ridge of femur			Plantarflexes ankle and provides proprioceptive information on tension of triceps surae
Popliteus	Lateral femoral condyle and lateral meniscus	Tibia		Flexes and unlocks knee

(continued)

Muscles of the leg *(continued)*

Muscle	Proximal Attachment	Distal Attachment	Innervation	Main Actions
Tibialis posterior	Fibula and interosseous membrane	Tuberosity of navicular		Plantarflexes ankle, inverts foot
Flexor hallucis longus		Distal phalanx digit 1		Flexes joints of 1st digit, plantarflexes ankle, and supports longitudinal arches of foot
Flexor digitorum longus	Tibia and fibula	Distal phalanges digits 2–5		Plantarflexes ankle, flexes digits 2–5, and supports longitudinal arches of foot

Additional Concept

Triceps Surae

The gastrocnemius, soleus, and plantaris are collectively referred to as the **triceps surae**.

Clinical Significance

Compartment Syndrome

Compartment syndrome is increased intracompartment pressure due to muscle swelling or **shin splints**. Shin splints is pain resulting from repetitive microtrauma to the tibialis anterior.

Gastrocnemius

Gastrocnemius strain is a painful injury resulting from tearing the medial belly of the muscle during knee extension and dorsiflexion of the ankle.

Mnemonics

Eversion versus Inversion

The second letter in the name of the muscle indicates the function:

Eversion:
perineus longus
perineus brevis

perineus tertius
Inversion:
tibialis anterior
tibialis posterior

Plantarflexion

Plantarflexion occurs when you step on a **plant** with the sole of your foot.

Nerves of the leg

Nerve	Origin	Structures Innervated
Tibial	Sciatic	Supplies gastrocnemius, soleus, plantaris, popliteus, flexor hallucis longus, flexor digitorum longus, and tibialis posterior
Common fibular		Gives rise to the lateral sural cutaneous and superficial and deep fibular
Superficial fibular	Common fibular	Supplies fibularis longus and brevis and sensory to anterior aspect of distal leg
Deep fibular		Supplies tibialis anterior, extensor hallucis longus, extensor digitorum longus, and fibularis tertius
Posterior femoral cutaneous	Sacral plexus	Sensory to skin of calf
Saphenous	Femoral	• Sensory to medial aspect of leg • Runs with great saphenous vein
Lateral sural cutaneous	Common fibular	Sensory to posterolateral aspect of leg
Medial sural cutaneous	Tibial	Sensory to posterior aspect of leg
Superficial fibular	Common fibular	Sensory to anterolateral aspect of leg
Sural	Common fibular and tibial	Sensory to lateral and posterior aspect of leg

Vessels of the leg
(Figure 5-2)

Artery	Origin	Description
Popliteal	Femoral	• Begins at the adductor hiatus as a continuation of the femoral • Gives rise to genicular, anterior, and posterior tibial arteries
Genicular	Popliteal	• Composed of superior lateral and medial, inferior lateral, and medial genicular • Contribute the anastomosis around the knee joint

(continued)

Vessels of the leg *(continued)*

Artery	Origin	Supplies/Gives Rise to
Anterior tibial		• Runs with deep fibular nerve on interosseous membrane • Supplies anterior leg and dorsum of foot, terminates as the dorsalis pedis
Posterior tibial		• Gives off fibular artery • Supplies posterior aspect of leg and sole of foot, terminates as medial and lateral plantar arteries
Fibular	Posterior tibial	Supplies posterolateral aspects of leg

Additional Concept

Venous Drainage

Venous drainage generally parallels arterial supply.

Clinical Significance

Posterior Tibial Artery

The **posterior tibial arterial** pulse can be palpated between the medial malleolus and the calcaneal tendon.

FOOT REGION

Bones of the foot
(Figures 5-1 and 5-4)

Bone	Characteristic	Significance
Talus	Trochlea	Articulates with tibia and malleoli of tibia and fibula
	Head	Articulates with the navicular, forming a ball-and-socket type joint, supported inferiorly by the plantar calcaneonavicular ligament
Cal-caneus	Calcaneal tuberosity	Attachment for abductor digiti minimi, abductor hallucis, flexor digitorum brevis, plantar aponeurosis, long plantar ligament, quadratus plantae, and the plantar calcaneo-cuboid ligament
	Fibular trochlea	Separates grooves for the tendons of fibularis longus and brevis

(continued)

Bones of the foot *(continued)*

Bone	Characteristic	Significance
	Talar shelf	Attachment for tibialis posterior, deltoid ligament, and plantar calcaneonavicular ligament; inferior surface grooved for tendon of flexor hallucis longus
Navicular	Tuberosity	Attachment for tibialis posterior
Cuboid		Bears facet for sesamoid bone in tendon of fibularis longus to glide
Medial cuneiform	Articular surfaces	Articulates with 4 bones—navicular, intermediate cuneiform, and 1st and 2nd metatarsals
Intermediate cuneiform		Articulates with 4 bones—navicular, medial and lateral cuneiforms, and 2nd metatarsal
Lateral cuneiform		Articulates with 6 bones—navicular, intermediate cuneiform, cuboid, and 2nd, 3rd, 4th metatarsals
Metatarsals (5)	Base	Articulate with tarsal bones and adjacent metatarsals
Proximal phalanges (5)	Heads	Articulate with proximal phalanges
Middle phalanges (5)		Articulate with more distal phalanges
Distal phalanges (4)	Tuberosity	Ungual tuberosity supports the toenail

Clinical Significance

Avulsion

Sudden inversion of the foot may cause avulsion of the tuberosity of the **5th metatarsal,** the attachment for fibularis brevis.

Muscles of the foot

Muscle	Proximal Attachment	Distal Attachment	Innervation	Main Actions
Dorsum				
Extensor digitorum brevis	Calcaneus	Tendons of extensor digitorum longus	Deep fibular	Extend digits 2–5

(continued)

Muscles of the foot *(continued)*

Muscle	Proximal Attachment	Distal Attachment	Innervation	Main Actions
Extensor hallucis brevis		Proximal phalanx of digit 1		Extend digit 1
Plantar Surface—Layer 1 (Most Superficial)				
Abductor hallucis	Calcaneus	Proximal phalanx of digit 1	Medial plantar	Abducts digit 1
Flexor digitorum brevis		Middle phalanges of digits 2–5		Flexes middle phalanges of digits 2–5
Abductor digiti minimi		Proximal phalanx of digit 5	Lateral plantar	Abducts digit 5
Plantar Surface—Layer 2				
Quadratus plantae	Calcaneus	Tendons of flexor digitorum longus	Lateral plantar	Assists with toe flexion
Lumbricals	Tendons of flexor digitorum longus	Extensor expansions	• 1st: medial plantar • 2nd–4th: lateral plantar	Flex metatarsophalangeal joints, extend interphalangeal joints
Plantar Surface—Layer 3				
Flexor hallucis brevis	Cuboid and 3rd cuneiform	Proximal phalanx of digit 1	Medial plantar	Flexes digit 1
Adductor hallucis	• Oblique head: metatarsals 2–4 • Traverse head: metatarsophalangeal joints		Lateral plantar	• Adducts digit 1 • Maintains transverse arch of foot
Flexor digiti minimi brevis	5th metatarsal	Proximal phalanx of digit 5		Flexes digit 5
Plantar Surface—Layer 4				
Plantar interossei (3)	Metatarsals 3–5	Proximal phalanges 3–5	Lateral plantar	• Adducts digits 2–4 • Flex metatarsophalangeal joints
Dorsal interossei (4)	Metatarsals 1–5	Proximal phalanges 2–4		• Abducts digits 2–4 • Flex metatarsophalangeal joints

Clinical Significance

Extensor Digitorum Brevis

A hematoma resulting from trauma to the **extensor digitorum brevis** produces edema near the ankle that is often confused with an ankle sprain.

Nerves of the foot

Nerve	Origin	Structures Innervated
Saphenous	Femoral	• Runs with great saphenous vein • Sensory to medial aspect of foot
Medial sural cutaneous	Tibial	Sensory to lateral aspect of ankle and foot
Superficial fibular	Common fibular	Sensory to dorsum of foot
Deep fibular		• Supplies extensor digitorum brevis • Sensory to skin between the 1st and 2nd toes
Calcaneal(s)	Tibial and sural	Sensory to heel
Medial plantar	Tibial	• Supplies abductor hallucis, flexor digitorum brevis, flexor hallucis brevis and 1st lumbrical • Sensory to medial aspect of sole and medial 3½ toes
Lateral plantar		• Supplies quadratus planate, abductor digiti minimi, flexor digiti minimi brevis, plantar and dorsal interossei, lateral 3 lumbricals, and adductor hallucis • Sensory to lateral aspect of sole and lateral 1½ toes
Sural	Tibial and common fibular	Sensory to lateral aspect of foot

Vessels of the foot
(Figure 5-2)

Artery	Origin	Description
Dorsal Surface		
Dorsalis pedis	Anterior tibial	• Continuation of the anterior tibial after it passes into the foot • Gives rise to the lateral tarsal, arcuate, 1st dorsal metatarsal, and deep plantar
Lateral tarsal	Dorsalis pedis	Anastomosis with arcuate
Arcuate		Gives the 2nd, 3rd, and 4th dorsal metatarsals

(continued)

Vessels of the foot *(continued)*

Artery	Origin	Description
Dorsal metatarsals	Arcuate	Give off 2 dorsal digitals
Dorsal digitals	Dorsal metatarsals	Supplies the digits
1st dorsal metatarsal	Dorsalis pedis	Supplies the 1st digit
Deep plantar		Anastomosis with lateral plantar to form plantar arch
Plantar Surface		
Medial plantar	Posterior tibial	Divides into superficial and deep branches that supply the digits
Lateral plantar		Forms plantar arch with deep plantar
Plantar metatarsals	Plantar arch	Give rise to plantar digitals
Plantar digitals	Plantar metatarsals	Supply the digits
Plantar arch	Lateral plantar	Gives rise to plantar metatarsals

Additional Concept

Venous Drainage

Venous drainage generally parallels arterial supply.

MISCELLANEOUS

Areas of lower limb
(Figure 5-3)

Feature	Structure	Significance
Femoral triangle	Triangular region in antero-superior aspect of thigh, deep to fascia lata: • Superior border (base): inguinal ligament • Medial border: adductor longus • Lateral border: sartorius • Roof: fascia lata—deficiency: cribriform fascia and saphenous opening, pierced by great saphenous vein • Floor: iliopsoas (laterally) and pectineus (medially)	Location of neurovascular structures entering and leaving thigh through subinguinal space, from lateral to medial: • Femoral nerve • Femoral sheath—contains: • Femoral artery • Femoral vein • Femoral canal (fat and deep inguinal lymph nodes)

(continued)

Areas of lower limb *(continued)*

Feature	Structure	Significance
Adductor canal	• Intermuscular passage found deep to sartorius • Proximal opening—apex of femoral triangle, distal opening—adductor hiatus	• Also known as subsartorial canal • Transmits femoral artery, femoral vein, and saphenous nerve
Popliteal fossa	Fat-filled, diamond-shaped space posterior to knee joint; boundaries: • Superolateral: biceps femoris • Superomedial: semimembra-nosus • Inferolateral: gastrocnemius • Inferomedial: gastrocnemius • Roof: popliteal fascia • Floor: popliteus	Contains: • Popliteal artery • Popliteal vein—receives small saphenous vein in fossa • Tibial nerve • Common fibular nerve • Popliteal lymph nodes
Arches of the foot	3 arches formed by bones, muscles, tendons, ligaments, and fascia 1. Medial longitudinal arch 2. Lateral longitudinal arch 3. Transverse arch	• Act as shock absorbers and springboards during locomotion and bear weight of body • Maintained by passive and dynamic support: 　• **Passive**—bones, connective tissue structures (plantar aponeurosis and long, short and spring ligaments) 　• **Dynamic**—intrinsic muscles of foot and tendons of leg muscles passing into foot

Mnemonics

Borders of Popliteal Fossa

The two "semi" muscles go together—semimembranosus and semitendinosus.

Semi contains an "M"; therefore, they are medial, leaving biceps femoris as the lateral border.

Borders of Femoral Triangle

So I May Always Love Sally:
Superior: Inguinal ligament
Medial: Adductor longus
Lateral: Sartorius

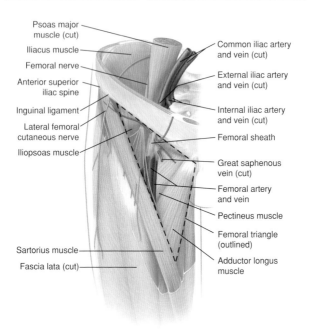

FIGURE 5-3. Femoral triangle, anterior view. (From Tank PW, Gest TR. *LWW Atlas of Anatomy.* Baltimore: Lippincott Williams & Wilkins; 2009:104.)

Contents of Femoral Triangle

NAVEL
femoral Nerve
femoral Artery
femoral Vein
Empty space, containing
Lymphatics

Clinical Significance

Femoral Ring

The "empty space" of the mnemonic is the femoral canal; the proximal opening of the femoral canal is the **femoral ring**, a common site for a femoral hernia.

Superficial structures of the lower limb

Structure	Course/Significance
Vessel	
Great saphenous vein	• Origin: dorsal digital vein of 1st digit and the dorsal venous arch • Runs anterior to medial malleolus, posterior to medial femoral condyle • Passes through saphenous opening to enter femoral vein
Small saphenous vein	• Origin: dorsal digital vein of 5th digit and the dorsal venous arch • Runs posterior to lateral malleolus superiorly along posterior aspect of the leg • Pierces the deep fascia to enter the popliteal vein in the popliteal fossa
Dorsal venous arch	Highly variable superficial venous network on dorsum of foot
Perforating veins	Drain venous blood from superficial veins to deep veins
Lymphatics of lower limb	Superficial lymphatic vessels accompany veins to enter superficial lymph nodes, including popliteal, inguinal, and external iliac groups
Cutaneous Nerve	
Subcostal	• Origin: T12 • Lateral cutaneous branch is sensory to skin of hip
Genitofemoral	• Origin: lumbar plexus • Sensory to skin of femoral triangle
Iliohypogastric	• Origin: lumbar plexus • Lateral cutaneous branch is sensory to skin of supero-lateral gluteal region
Ilioinguinal	• Origin: lumbar plexus • Femoral branch is sensory to skin of femoral triangle
Lateral cutaneous nerve of thigh	• Origin: lumbar plexus • Sensory to skin of lateral and anterior thigh
Obturator	Cutaneous branch sensory to skin of medial aspect of thigh
Femoral	Cutaneous branch sensory to skin of anterior and medial thigh
Saphenous	• Origin: femoral • Sensory to skin of medial aspect of leg • Runs with great saphenous vein
Lateral sural cutaneous	• Origin: common fibular • Sensory to skin of posterolateral leg
Medial sural cutaneous	• Origin: tibial • Sensory to skin of posterior leg and lateral ankle and foot
Sural	• Origin: tibial and common fibular • Sensory to skin of posterolateral leg

(continued)

Superficial structures of the lower limb *(continued)*

Structure	Course/Significance
Superficial fibular	• Origin: common fibular • Sensory to skin of anterolateral leg and dorsal aspect of foot
Deep fibular	• Origin: common fibular • Sensory to skin between the 1st and 2nd digit on the dorsum of the foot
Clunials	• Superior, middle, and inferior • Origin: lumbar and sacral plexuses and branches of the posterior cutaneous nerve of the thigh • Sensory to skin of gluteal region
Posterior cutaneous nerve of thigh	• Origin: sacral plexus • Sensory to skin of posterior aspect of thigh
Lateral plantar	• Origin: tibial • Sensory to skin of lateral aspect of sole of foot
Medial plantar	• Origin: tibial • Sensory to skin of medial aspect of sole of foot
Tibial	Calcaneal branches are sensory to skin over calcaneus

Clinical Significance

Nerve Block

The ilioinguinal and iliohypogastric nerves can be blocked by injecting anesthetic near the anterior superior iliac spine; the femoral can be blocked near the midpoint of the inguinal ligament.

Great Saphenous Vein

The great saphenous vein and its tributaries may become varicose, mainly from incompetent valves. During saphenous cutdown, an incision is made anterior to the medial malleolus to locate the great saphenous vein for infusion of therapeutic agents.

Fascia of lower limb

Fascia/ Connective Tissue	Significance/Structure
Fascia lata	Deep fascia of the thigh
Iliotibial tract	• Thickening of fascia lata over lateral aspect of thigh • Extends from iliac tubercle to lateral condyle of tibia • Attachment for tensor fascia lata and gluteus maximus

(continued)

Fascia of lower limb (continued)

Fascia/Connective Tissue	Significance/Structure
Saphenous opening	• Hiatus in the fascia lata inferior to the medial aspect of inguinal ligament • Falciform margin (lateral and inferior) is sharp • Covered by cribriform fascia • Great saphenous vein passes through to enter femoral vein
Falciform margin	Sharp inferior and lateral borders of saphenous opening
Cribriform fascia	Membranous layer of subcutaneous tissue that covers the saphenous opening
Crural fascia	Deep fascia of the leg
Extensor retinacula	Thickened crural fascia over distal leg
Femoral sheath	• Extension of transversalis fascia through subinguinal space into the femoral triangle • Divided into 3 compartments that transmit femoral artery, vein, and femoral canal between the abdominopelvic cavity and femoral triangle of the thigh
Femoral canal	• Medial-most of the 3 compartments of the femoral sheath • Contains fat and lymphatics • Allows for expansion of femoral vein during increased venous return
Popliteal fascia	Deep fascia forming roof of popliteal fossa
Plantar fascia	• Deep fascia of sole of foot • Thickened central aspect forms plantar aponeurosis • Protects sole of foot and supports arches
Plantar aponeurosis	• Thickened central region of plantar fascia • Reinforced distally by superficial transverse metatarsal ligament • Vertical septa extend superiorly from aponeurosis to divide foot into 3 compartments: 1. Medial 2. Central 3. Lateral

Additional Concept

Fourth Compartment

Distally, a fourth compartment—the interosseous compartment of the foot exists.

Clinical Significance

Compartment Syndrome

Increased pressure in the fascial compartments of the lower limb produces compartment syndromes, causing pain and tissue damage.

Plantar Fasciitis

Inflammation of the **plantar aponeurosis**—plantar fasciitis, results from high-impact exercise and causes pain over the heel and medial aspects of the foot.

Lumbosacral plexus

Nerve	Significance/Structure
Roots	L1–S4 spinal nerves' anterior rami form plexus
Divisions	Rami terminate by dividing into an anterior and posterior divisions
Branches (6): 1. Femoral nerve 2. Obturator nerve 3. Common fibular nerve 4. Tibial nerve 5. Superior gluteal nerve 6. Inferior gluteal nerve	1. Femoral nerve (L2–L4) 2. Obturator nerve (L2–L4) 3. Common fibular nerve (L4–S2; terminates by dividing into superficial and deep fibular nerves) 4. Tibial nerve (L4–S3) • 1–4 above innervate the lower limb 5. Superior gluteal nerve (L4–S1) 6. Inferior gluteal nerve (L5–S2) • 5–6 above innervate the gluteal region • The common fibular and tibial nerves comprise the sciatic nerve

Clinical Significance

Femoral Nerve

Injury to the **femoral nerve** results in the loss of leg extension and therefore loss of the knee jerk reflex.

Common Fibular Nerve

Loss of dorsiflexion and eversion of the foot as a result of **common fibular nerve** damage leads to foot drop and foot slap.

Superior Gluteal Nerve

Injury to the **superior gluteal nerve** results in paralysis of gluteus medius and minimus, resulting in the inability to steady the pelvis during walking, leading to a positive Trendelenburg sign and a waddling gait.

Inferior Gluteal Nerve

Paralysis of the gluteus maximus, as occurs with injury to the **inferior gluteal nerve** results in weakness when extending the thigh/hip, leading to difficulty rising from a seated position and climbing stairs.

Joints of lower limb
(Figure 5-5)

Joint	Type	Articulation	Structure	Movements
Hip	Synovial	Head of femur with acetabulum	• Iliofemoral (anterior), pubofemoral (inferior), and ischio-femoral (posterior) ligaments support joint • Acetabular labrum and transverse acetabular ligament deepen socket • Ligamentum teres carries the artery to the head of the femur	Flexion, extension, abduction, adduction, medial rotation, lateral rotation, and circum-duction
Femoro-tibial (knee)		Medial and lateral femoral condyles with medial and lateral condy-les of tibia	• 5 extracap-sular liga-ments: 1. Patellar 2. Fibular collateral 3. Tibial collateral 4. Oblique popliteal 5. Arcuate popliteal • 4 intra-articular ligaments/ structures: 1. Anterior cruciate	Flexion, extension, medial rotation, and lateral rotation

(continued)

Joint	Type	Articulation	Structure	Movements
			2. Posterior cruciate 3. Medial menisci 4. Lateral menisci • Popliteus tendon strengthens the joint	
Superior tibiofibular and tibio-fibular syn-desmosis (inferior)	• Superior: synovial • Inferior: fibrous	• Superior: head of fibula with tibial condyle • Inferior: fibula with tibia	• Superior: anterior and posterior ligaments of the head of the fibula strengthen joint capsule • Inferior: interosseous membrane and anterior and posterior tibiofibular and inferior transverse tibiofibular ligament strengthen joint	Small amount of movement during dorsiflexion
Talocrural (ankle)	Synovial	Medial malle-olus and distal end of tibia and lateral malleolus of fibula with the trochlea of the talus	• Lateral ligament: calcaneo-fibular, an-terior, and posterior talofibular • Medial (deltoid) ligament: anterior and posterior tibiotalar, tibionavicu-lar, and tibio-calcaneal strengthen and stabilize joint	Dorsiflexion, plantarflexion

(continued)

Joints of lower limb *(continued)*

Joint	Type	Articulation	Structure	Movements
Talocal-caneal (subtalar)		Inferior surface of talus with superior surface of calcaneus	• Interosseous talocalca-neal liga-ment binds bodies of calcaneus and talus • Medial, lateral, and posterior talocalca-neal liga-ment sup-ports joint	Inversion, eversion
Intertarsal (talocal-caneona-vicular, calcaneo-cuboid, cuneona-vicular)		Between ad-jacent tarsal bones	Ligaments, named for the bones they connect, support joint	Mainly gliding movements
Tarsome-tatarsal		Distal tarsal bones with proximal end of metatarsals	Interosseous tarsometarsal, dorsal, and plantar liga-ments streng-then joint	Gliding
Metatar-sophalan-geal		Head of meta-tarsals with proximal phalanges	Plantar and collateral ligaments support joint	Flexion, extension, abduction, adduction, and circumduction
Interpha-langeal		Heads of proximal phalanges articulate with more distal phalanges	Plantar and collateral ligaments support joint	Flexion, extension

Additional Concept

The inferior tibiofibular joint is the inferiormost part of the tibiofibular syndesmosis.

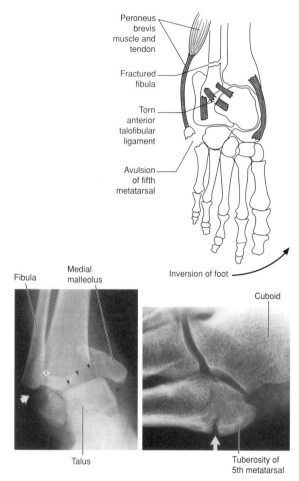

FIGURE 5-4. Inversion injury. Inversion injuries are more common owing to the strength of the deltoid ligament (medial collateral) on the medial side of the ankle; they are most likely to occur during dorsiflexion, when the ankle is most unstable. (From Dudek RW, Louis TM. *High-Yield Gross Anatomy.* 3rd ed. Baltimore: Lippincott Williams & Wilkins; 2008:256.)

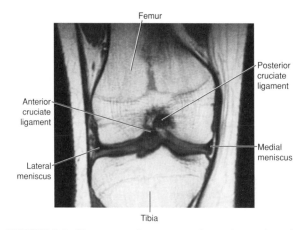

FIGURE 5-5. Knee magnetic resonance image (coronal section through the intercondylar notch). (From Dudek RW, Louis TM. *High-Yield Gross Anatomy.* 3rd ed. Baltimore: Lippincott Williams & Wilkins; 2008:253.)

Clinical Significance

Hip Dislocation

Congenital dislocation of the hip joint is common, particularly in girls.

Knee Injuries

Anterior cruciate ligament rupture allows the tibia to slide anteriorly relative to the femur—anterior drawer sign; posterior cruciate ligament rupture allows the tibia to slide posteriorly relative to the femur—posterior drawer sign.

Mnemonic

Structures Posterior to Medial Malleolus

From anterior to posterior—Tom, Dick And Very Nervous Harry

Tibialis posterior
extensor Digitorum longus
posterior tibial Artery
posterior tibial Vein
tibial Nerve

6

Upper Limb

INTRODUCTION

The upper limb is divided for descriptive purposes by skeletal elements into:

- shoulder—portion between the arm and the thorax that includes the pectoral girdle: scapula and clavicle
- arm—portion between the shoulder and elbow that includes the humerus
- forearm—portion between the elbow and wrist that includes the radius and ulna
- hand—portion distal to the wrist that includes the metacarpals and phalanges, the carpal bones form the wrist

SHOULDER REGION

Bones of the shoulder
(Figure 6-1)

Bone	Feature	Significance
Clavicle	Shaft	• S-shaped, serves as strut to suspend limb away from body • Protects neurovascular bundle serving upper limb • Attachment for pectoralis major—clavicular head, sternocleidomastoid—clavicular head, trapezius, subclavius, and deltoid
	Acromial end	Articulates with the acromion of the scapula at acromioclavicular joint
	Sternal end	Articulates with the manubrium of the sternum at sternoclavicular joint
Scapula	Spine	• Divides posterior aspect of scapula into supra- and infraspinous fossae • Attachment for trapezius and deltoid

(continued)

Bones of the shoulder *(continued)*

Bone	Feature	Significance
	Supraspinous fossa	Attachment for supraspinatus
	Infraspinous fossa	Attachment for infraspinatus
	Subscapular fossa	Attachment for subscapularis
	Acromion	• Expanded, lateral end of spine, forms "point" of the shoulder • Articulates with acromial end of clavicle • Attachment for trapezius and deltoid
	Glenoid fossa	• Articulates with head of humerus at glenohumeral joint • Deepened by glenoid labrum
	Supraglenoid tubercle	Attachment for long head of biceps brachii
	Infraglenoid tubercle	Attachment for long head of triceps brachii
	Coracoid process	• Attachment for biceps brachii (short head), coracobrachialis, and pectoralis minor muscles • Attachment for coracoclavicular and coracoacromial ligaments and the costocoracoid membrane
	Suprascapular notch	• Transmits the suprascapular nerve • Bridged by the superior transverse scapular ligament • The omohyoid attaches medial to the notch
	Inferior angle	Attachment for teres major and serratus anterior
	Medial border	Attachment for levator scapulae, rhomboids (major and minor) and serratus anterior
	Superior angle	Attachment for levator scapulae
	Lateral border	Attachment for teres minor

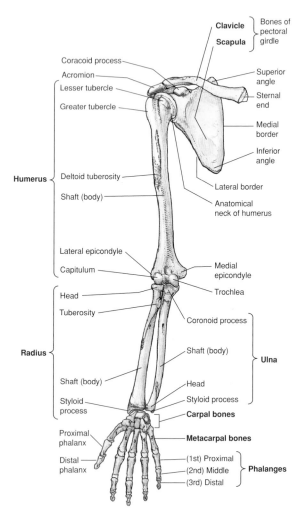

FIGURE 6-1. All bones, upper limb, anterior view. The right superior appendicular skeleton includes the right half of the pectoral (shoulder) girdle, composed of the right clavicle and scapula, and the skeleton of the free right upper limb, formed by the remaining bones distal to the scapula. (From Moore KL, Dalley AF. *Clinically Oriented Anatomy.* 5th ed. Baltimore: Lippincott Williams & Wilkins; 2006:728.)

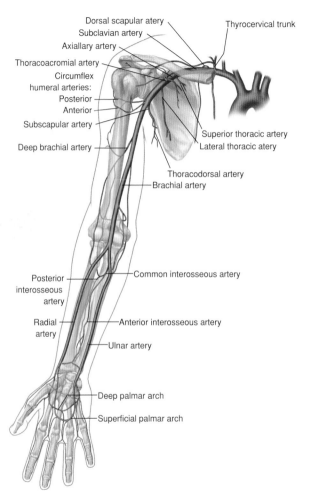

FIGURE 6-2. Arteries of upper limb, anterior view. (From Tank PW, Gest TR. *LWW Atlas of Anatomy*. Baltimore: Lippincott Williams & Wilkins; 2009:75.)

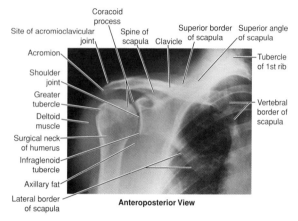

Anteroposterior View

FIGURE 6-3. Shoulder bone radiograph. (From Dudek RW, Louis TM. *High-Yield Gross Anatomy.* 3rd ed. Baltimore: Lippincott Williams & Wilkins; 2008:230.)

Clinical Significance

Fractures

The **clavicle**, the first bone to begin ossification, is one of the most commonly fractured bones. Fracture is usually evident by the palpable elevation of the medial portion from action of the **sternocleidomastoid** and drooping of the shoulder from the unsupported weight of the upper limb.

Muscles of the shoulder

Muscle	Proximal Attachment	Distal Attachment	Innervation	Main Actions
Pectoralis major	• Clavicular head— medial half of clavicle • Sternal head— sternum, superior 6 costal cartilages	Lateral lip intertubercular groove of humerus	Medial and lateral pectorals	• Adducts, flexes, and medially rotates humerus • Draws scapula anteriorly

(continued)

Muscles of the shoulder *(continued)*

Muscle	Proximal Attachment	Distal Attachment	Innervation	Main Actions
	and external oblique aponeurosis			
Pectoralis minor	Ribs 3–5	Coracoid process of scapula	Medial pectoral	Stabilizes scapula
Serratus anterior	Ribs 1–8	Medial border of scapula	Long thoracic	• Protracts and rotates scapula • Holds scapula against thoracic wall
Subclavius	Junction of 1st rib and costal cartilage	Middle ⅓ of clavicle	Nerve to subclavius	Depresses clavicle
Trapezius	Superior nuchal line, external occipital protuberance, nuchal ligament, C7–C12 spinous processes	Lateral ⅓ of clavicle, acromion, spine, of scapula	Spinal accessory	• Elevation, depression, retraction of scapula • Rotates glenoid fossa superiorly
Latissimus dorsi	T6–T12 spinous processes, thoracolumbar fascia, iliac crest, and ribs 9–12	Floor of intertubercular groove of humerus	Thoracodorsal	Extends, adducts, medially rotates humerus
Levator scapulae	C1–C4 transverse processes	Medial border and superior angle of scapula	Dorsal scapular	Elevates scapula
Rhomboids—major and minor	• Major—T2–T5 spinous processes	• Major—medial border of scapula		

(continued)

Muscles of the shoulder *(continued)*

Muscle	Proximal Attachment	Distal Attachment	Innervation	Main Actions
	• Minor—nuchal ligament C7–T11 spinous processes	• Minor—spine of scapula		Retract and rotate scapula
Deltoid	• Clavicle • Acromion and spine of scapula	Deltoid tuberosity of humerus	Axillary	Flexes and medially rotates (anterior part), abducts (middle part), extends and laterally rotates (posterior part) arm
Supraspinatus	Supraspinous fossa of scapula	Greater tubercle of humerus	Suprascapular	• Initiates abduction of arm • Rotator cuff muscle
Infraspinatus	Infraspinous fossa of scapula			• Laterally rotates arm • Rotator cuff muscle
Teres minor	Lateral border of scapula		Axillary	
Teres major	Inferior angle of scapula	Medial lip of intertubercular groove of humerus	Lower subscapular	Adducts and medially rotates arm
Subscapularis	Subscapular fossa of scapula	Lesser tubercle of humerus	Upper and lower subscapular	• Adducts and medially rotates arm • Rotator cuff muscle

Clinical Significance

Serratus Anterior Paralysis

When **serratus anterior** is paralyzed owing to injury of the **long thoracic nerve**, the medial border moves laterally and posteriorly away from the thoracic wall, giving the scapula the appearance of a wing—**winged scapula**.

Mnemonics

Long Thoracic Nerve

C5–C7, raise your wings to heaven.
C5–C7 (cord levels found within the serratus anterior)
  injury causes inability to "raise" arm past 90 degrees
  (to heaven) and results in a winged scapula.
SALT—**S**erratus **A**nterior; **L**ong **T**horacic nerve

Rotator Cuff

The humeral head **SITS** in the glenoid fossa because of the
rotator cuff muscles—**S**upraspinatus, **I**nfraspinatus, **T**eres
Minor, **S**ubscapularis.

Nerves of the shoulder

Nerve	Origin	Structures Innervated
Supraclavicular nerves	Cervical plexus (C3–C4)	Sensory to skin of shoulder
Axillary	Posterior cord	Teres minor, shoulder joint, deltoid, skin of shoulder
Dorsal scapular	C5	Rhomboids, levator scapulae
Spinal accessory (CN XI)	1st few cervical spinal cord segments	Trapezius and sternocleidomastoid

Clinical Significance

Axillary Nerve

The **deltoid** atrophies when the **axillary nerve** is damaged,
as happens during fracture of the surgical neck of the
humerus or inferior dislocation of the **glenohumeral joint**.
A loss of sensation over the proximal arm accompanies atro-
phy of the deltoid.

Vessels of the shoulder
(Figure 6-2)

Artery	Origin	Description
Subclavian— right and left	• Right— brachiocephalic trunk • Left—arch of the aorta	• Ends at lateral border of 1st rib to become the axillary • Gives rise to vertebral, internal thoracic, and thyrocervical trunk

(continued)

Vessels of the shoulder *(continued)*

Artery	Origin	Description
Internal thoracic	1st part of subclavian	Gives rise to anterior intercostals, musculophrenic, superior epigastric, and pericardiacophrenic
Thyrocervical trunk		Gives rise to suprascapular, transverse cervical, inferior thyroid, and ascending cervical
Suprascapular	Thyrocervical trunk	Supplies shoulder region
Transverse cervical		
Axillary	Subclavian at lateral border of 1st rib	• 1st part—superior thoracic • 2nd part—thoracoacromial, lateral thoracic • 3rd part—anterior humeral circumflex, posterior humeral circumflex, and subscapular
Superior thoracic	1st part of axillary	Supplies 1st and 2nd intercostal spaces, serratus anterior
Thoracoacromial	2nd part of axillary	Gives rise to pectoral, deltoid, acromial, and clavicular branches
Lateral thoracic		Supplies lateral aspect of breast
Circumflex humeral (anterior and posterior)	3rd part of axillary	Supplies area around neck of humerus
Subscapular		Gives rise to circumflex scapular and thoracodorsal
Circumflex scapular	Subscapular	Supplies scapular region
Thoracodorsal		Supplies latissimus dorsi

Additional Concept

Venous Drainage

Venous drainage generally parallels arterial supply.

Clinical Significance

Axillary Artery

The **axillary artery** can be compressed against the **humerus** or the first rib if profuse bleeding occurs. Branches of the axillary artery contribute to the extensive anastomoses around the scapula, which may serve to protect the limb during occlusion or compression of the primary arterial pathways.

Aneurysm of the axillary artery may compress the **trunks** of the **brachial plexus,** leading to pain and anesthesia in the areas supplied by the affected nerves.

Mnemonics

Axillary Artery Branches

The axillary artery is divided into three parts by the pectoralis minor. The parts correspond to the number of branches:

1. Part 1—proximal to pectoralis minor has one branch: superior thoracic
2. Part 2—deep to pectoralis minor has two branches: thoracoacromial and lateral thoracic arteries
3. Part 3—distal to pectoralis minor has three branches: anterior and posterior humeral circumflex and the subscapular trunk

Send The Lord to Say A Prayer—proximal to distal branches off of the axillary artery:

Superior Thoracic
Thoracoacromial
Lateral Thoracic
Subscapular
Anterior Circumflex Humeral
Posterior Circumflex Humeral

Thoracoacromial Trunk Branches

CAlifornia Police Department—branches of the thoracoacromial trunk:
Clavicular
Acromial
Pectoral
Deltoid

ARM REGION

Bones of the arm
(Figures 6-1, 6-3, and 6-7)

Bone	Characteristic	Significance
Humerus	Head	Articulates with glenoid fossa of the scapula to form glenohumeral joint

(continued)

Bones of the arm *(continued)*

Bone	Characteristic	Significance
	Greater tubercle	• Lateral aspect of humerus • Attachment for supraspinatus, infraspinatus, and teres minor
	Lesser tubercle	• Medial aspect of humerus • Attachment for subscapularis
	Anatomical neck	Attachment for glenohumeral joint capsule
	Surgical neck	• Common site for humeral fracture • Distal to greater and lesser tubercles • Axillary nerve and posterior humeral circumflex artery are found nearby and are subject to injury during fracture at the neck
	Intertubercular groove (bicipital groove)	• Located between the greater and lesser tubercles • Transmits tendon of the long head of the biceps brachii • Bridged by the transverse humeral ligament • Lateral lip attachment for pectoralis major • Floor attachment for latissimus dorsi • Medial lip attachment for teres major
	Lateral epicondyle	Attachment for common extensor tendon of the forearm and the supinator
	Medial epicondyle	Attachment for common flexor tendon of the forearm and pronator teres
	Lateral supracondylar ridge	Attachment for brachioradialis, extensor carpi radialis longus and medial head of triceps brachii
	Medial supracondylar ridge	Attachment for brachialis and the medial head of triceps brachii
	Trochlea	Articulates with trochlear notch of ulna
	Capitulum	Articulates with head of radius
	Radial fossa	Receives the head of the radius during forearm flexion
	Olecranon fossa	Receives olecranon of the ulna during forearm extension
	Coronoid fossa	Receives coronoid process of ulna during forearm flexion

(continued)

Bones of the arm *(continued)*

Bone	Characteristic	Significance
	Radial (spiral) groove	• Transmits the deep brachial artery and radial nerve • Separates the proximal attachments of the lateral head (lateral to groove) and medial head (medial to groove) of the triceps brachii
	Deltoid tuberosity	Attachment for deltoid

Mnemonic

Intertubercular Groove Muscle Attachments

The lady between two majors.

Teres **major** attaches to the medial lip of the intertubercular groove.

Pectoralis **major** attaches to the lateral lip of the intertubercular groove.

Lati**ss**imus (lady) Dorsi attaches to the floor of the groove, between the two majors.

Clinical Significance

Fractures

Most humeral fractures occur at the **surgical neck**, resulting in an impacted fracture. A fall on the **acromion** may result in an avulsion fracture in which the **greater tubercle** is pulled away from the humerus. A direct blow to the arm may result in a transverse or spiral fracture of the shaft, whereas an intercondylar fracture may occur during a fall on a flexed **elbow**.

Muscles of the arm

Muscle	Proximal Attachment	Distal Attachment	Innervation	Main Actions
Coraco-brachialis	Coracoid process	Humerus	Musculocutaneous	Flexes and adducts arm
Biceps brachii	• Long head—supraglenoid tubercle • Short head—coracoid process	Radial tuberosity	Musculocutaneous	Flexes arm and forearm, supinates
Brachialis	Distal humerus, including medial supracondylar ridge	Ulnar tuberosity	Musculocutaneous	Flexes forearm

(continued)

Muscles of the arm *(continued)*

Muscle	Proximal Attachment	Distal Attachment	Innervation	Main Actions
Triceps brachii	• Long head—infraglenoid tubercle • Lateral head—lateral to radial groove • Medial head—medial to radial groove, medial and lateral supracondylar ridges	Olecranon process	Radial	Extends forearm
Anconeus	Lateral epicondyle	Olecranon process	Radial	Extends forearm

Mnemonic

Biceps Brachii Attachments

You ride **shorter** to the street **corner** and ride **longer** on the **super**highway.—

Short head of the biceps brachii attaches to the **coracoid** process.

Long head of the biceps brachii attaches to the **supraglenoid** tubercle.

Clinical Significance

Tendonitis of the Biceps Brachii

Biceps tendonitis, inflammation of the tendon of the **long head**, is the result of repetitive movement of the tendon in the **intertubercular groove**, as occurs in sports that involve throwing. Rupture of the tendon may occur as the tendon is torn from the **supraglenoid tubercle**.

Nerves of the arm

Nerve	Origin	Structures Innervated
Dorsal scapular	C5	Rhomboids, levator scapulae
Long thoracic	Superior trunk	Serratus anterior
Suprascapular		Supraspinatus and infraspinatus
Nerve to subclavius		Subclavius

(continued)

Nerves of the arm *(continued)*

Nerve	Origin	Structures Innervated
Lateral pectoral	Lateral cord	Pectoralis major
Musculocutaneous		• Anterior compartment of the arm • Sensory to lateral forearm
Median	Lateral cord and medial cord	• Anterior compartment of the forearm (except flexor carpi ulnaris and the ulnar half of flexor digitorum profundus), muscles of the thenar eminence and the first 2 lumbricals
Medial pectoral	Medial cord	Pectoralis minor and major
Ulnar		• Flexor carpi ulnaris and the ulnar half of flexor digitorum profundus • Most muscles of the hand • Sensory to hand medial to digit 4
Upper subscapular	Posterior cord	Subscapularis
Lower subscapular		Subscapularis and teres major
Thoracodorsal		Latissimus dorsi
Axillary		• Teres minor, deltoid • Shoulder joint, sensory to skin over shoulder
Radial		• Posterior compartments of arm and forearm • Sensory to skin of posterior arm, forearm, and hand

Clinical Significance

Thoracodorsal Nerve Injury

Injury to the **thoracodorsal nerve**, as may occur during resection of axillary lymph nodes in breast cancer, causes paralysis of the **latissimus dorsi**. The person is then unable to raise the trunk with the upper limbs or use an axillary crutch.

Arm vessels
(Figure 6-2)

Artery	Origin	Description
Axillary	Subclavian at lateral border of 1st rib	• 1st part—superior thoracic • 2nd part—thoracoacromial, lateral thoracic • 3rd part—anterior circumflex humeral, posterior circumflex humeral, and subscapular

(continued)

Arm vessels *(continued)*

Artery	Origin	Description
Circumflex humeral (anterior and posterior) arteries	3rd part of axillary	Supplies area around neck of humerus
Subscapular artery		Gives rise to circumflex scapular and thoracodorsal
Circumflex scapular artery	Subscapular	Supplies scapular region
Thoracodorsal artery		Supplies latissimus dorsi
Brachial artery	Axillary after lateral border of teres major	• Continuation of axillary • Terminates in elbow region to form radial and ulnar arteries
Deep brachial artery	Brachial	• Supplies posterior compartment of arm and elbow joint • Runs in radial groove with radial nerve
Superior ulnar collateral artery		Supplies elbow region
Inferior ulnar collateral artery		

Additional Concept
Venous Drainage
Venous drainage generally parallels arterial supply.

Clinical Significance
Brachial Artery
Compression of the **brachial artery** is best accomplished along the medial humerus in the mid-arm region. Collateral circulation through the deep brachial artery allows for perfusion distal to the compression.

FOREARM REGION

Bones of the forearm
(Figures 6-1 and 6-7)

Bone	Characteristic	Significance
Radius	Head	• Articulates with capitulum of humerus and radial notch of ulna • Held in place by the anular ligament
	Radial tuberosity	Attachment for biceps brachii
	Ulnar notch	Articulates with head of ulna
	Styloid process	Attachment for brachioradialis and radial collateral ligament
Ulna	Olecranon	Attachment for flexor carpi ulnaris (ulnar head), triceps brachii, anconeus, and ulnar collateral ligament
	Coronoid process	• Articulates with coronoid fossa of humerus during flexion • Attachment for pronator teres, flexor digitorum superficialis and ulnar collateral ligament
	Trochlear notch	Articulates with trochlea of humerus
	Ulnar tuberosity	Attachment for brachialis
	Radial notch	Articulates with head of radius
	Supinator crest	Attachment for supinator
	Supinator fossa	
	Head	Articulates with ulnar notch of radius and articular disc of the wrist
	Styloid process	Attachment for ulnar collateral ligament

Clinical Significance

Fractures

As a result of attempting to break a fall with the outstretched limb a **Colles' fracture** may occur. A Colles' fracture is a transverse fracture of the distal **radius**, often accompanied by an avulsed **styloid process** of the **ulna**. The result is a posterior angulation of the forearm, just proximal to the **wrist**—a dinner fork deformity.

Fractured Elbow

Fracture of the **olecranon**—a fractured elbow, is often caused by a fall. The **triceps brachii** pulls the avulsed piece of bone in this painful and debilitating injury.

Muscles of the forearm

Muscle	Proximal Attachment	Distal Attachment	Innervation	Main Actions
Pronator teres	Medial epicondyle of humerus and coronoid process of ulna	Mid-radius	Median	Pronates and flexes elbow
Flexor carpi radialis	Medial epicondyle of humerus	2nd metacarpal		Flexes wrist and abducts hand
Palmaris longus		Flexor retinaculum and palmar aponeurosis		Flexes wrist
Flexor carpi ulnaris	Medial epicondyle of humerus and olecranon process and posterior ulna	Pisiform, hook of hamate and 5th metacarpal	Ulnar	Flexes wrist and adducts hand
Flexor digitorum superficialis	Medial epicondyle of humerus and coronoid process of ulna and anterior radius	Middle phalanges of medial 4 digits	Median	Flexes proximal interphalangeal joints of medial 4 digits and flexes metacarpopha-langeal joints and flexes wrist
Flexor digitorum profundus	Ulna and interosseous membrane	Distal phalanges of medial 4 digits	Medial part—ulnar; lateral part—median	Flexes distal interphalangeal joints of medial 4 digits and flexes wrist
Flexor pollicis longus	Radius and interosseous membrane	Distal phalanx of thumb	Anterior interosseous (median)	Flexes thumb
Pronator quadratus	Ulna	Radius		Pronates
Brachiora-dialis	Lateral supracondylar ridge of humerus	Styloid process of radius	Radial	Flexes forearm
Extensor carpi radialis longus		2nd metacarpal		Extends hand and abducts wrist

(continued)

Muscles of the forearm *(continued)*

Muscle	Proximal Attachment	Distal Attachment	Innervation	Main Actions
Extensor carpi radialis brevis	Lateral epicondyle of humerus	3rd metacarpal	Deep radial (radial)	
Extensor digitorum		Extensor expansion of medial 4 digits	Posterior interosseous (radial)	Extends medial 4 digits
Extensor digiti minimi		5th digit extensor expansion		Extends 5th digit
Extensor carpi ulnaris	Lateral epicondyle of humerus and ulna	5th metacarpal		Extends hand and adducts wrist
Supinator	Lateral epicondyle of humerus, radial collateral ligament, anular ligament, supinator crest, and fossa of ulna	Proximal radius	Deep radial (radial)	Supinates
Abductor pollicis longus	Ulna, radius, and interosseous membrane	1st metacarpal	Posterior interosseous (radial)	Abducts thumb
Extensor pollicis longus	Ulna and interosseous membrane	Distal phalanx of thumb		Extends thumb
Extensor pollicis brevis	Radius and interosseous membrane	Proximal phalanx of thumb		
Extensor indicis	Ulna and interosseous membrane	2nd digit extensor expansion		Extends 2nd digit

Mnemonics

Relationship of Flexor Tendons in the Digits

Superficialis splits in two to permit profundus to pass through.

Relationship of Flexors in the Anterior Forearm

Tuck your thumb into your palm; lay your hand on your proximal forearm with the fingers pointed toward your hand. Your fingers represent the top layer of muscles:

2nd digit—pronator teres
3rd digit—flexor carpi radialis
4th digit—palmaris longus
5th digit—flexor carpi ulnaris

1st digit (thumb) represents the intermediate muscle layer—flexor digitorum superficialis

Clinical Significance

Elbow Tendonitis

Elbow tendonitis, or **tennis elbow**, is caused by repetitive use of the superficial extensor muscles of the forearm.

Forearm nerves

Nerve	Origin	Structures Innervated
Median	Union of lateral root (lateral cord) and medial root (medial cord)	Pronator teres, flexor carpi radialis, palmaris longus, and flexor digitorum superficialis
Anterior interosseous	Median	Lateral aspect of flexor digitorum profundus, flexor pollicis longus, and pronator quadratus
Ulnar	Medial cord of brachial plexus	Medial aspect of flexor digitorum profundus and flexor carpi ulnaris
Radial	Posterior cord of brachial plexus	Brachioradialis and extensor carpi radialis longus
Deep branch of radial	Radial	Extensor carpi radialis brevis, and supinator
Posterior interosseous	Deep branch of radial	Extensor digitorum, extensor digiti minimi, extensor carpi ulnaris, abductor pollicis longus, extensor pollicis longus, extensor pollicis brevis, and extensor indicis
Posterior cutaneous nerve of the forearm	Radial	Posterior aspect of the forearm

(continued)

Forearm nerves *(continued)*

Nerve	Origin	Structures Innervated
Lateral cutaneous nerve of the forearm	Musculocutaneous	Lateral aspect of the forearm
Medial cutaneous nerve of the forearm	Medial cord of brachial plexus	Medial aspect of the forearm

Mnemonic
Radial Nerve

The radial nerve innervates the **BEST** muscles—

Brachioradialis
Extensors
Supinator
Triceps Brachii

Vessels of the forearm
(Figure 6-2)

Artery	Origin	Description
Ulnar	Brachial	Terminal branch of the brachial
Radial		
Anterior ulnar recurrent	Ulnar	Supplies elbow region
Posterior ulnar recurrent		
Common interosseous		Gives rise to anterior and posterior interosseous
Anterior interosseous	Common interosseous	Supplies anterior aspect of forearm
Posterior interosseous		Supplies posterior aspect of forearm
Recurrent interosseous	Posterior interosseous	Supplies elbow region
Palmar carpal branch	Ulnar	Contributes to palmar carpal arch
Dorsal carpal branch		Contributes to dorsal carpal arch
Radial recurrent	Radial	Supplies elbow region
Palmar carpal branch		Contributes to palmar carpal arch
Dorsal carpal branch		Contributes to dorsal carpal arch

Additional Concept
Venous Drainage
Venous drainage generally parallels arterial supply.

Mnemonic

Arterial Anastomosis at Elbow

I Am Pretty Smart

Inferior ulnar collateral artery anastomoses with the Anterior ulnar recurrent artery. Posterior ulnar recurrent artery anastomoses with the Superior ulnar collateral artery.

HAND REGION

Bones of the hand
(Figures 6-1 and 6-4)

Bone	Characteristic	Significance
Scaphoid	Tubercle	• Attachment for abductor pollicis brevis, opponens pollicis, flexor pollicis brevis, radial collateral ligament, and flexor retinaculum (tubercle) • Articulates with radius, trapezium, lunate, capitate, and trapezoid • Most commonly fractured carpal bone
Lunate	Crescent-shaped	• Articulates with radius, scaphoid, triquetrum, capitate, and hamate • Most frequently dislocated carpal bone
Trique-trum	Pyramid-shaped	• Articulates with pisiform, hamate and lunate • Attachment for ulnar collateral ligament
Pisiform	Spheroidal	• Articulates with triquetrum • Attachment for flexor retinaculum, flexor carpi ulnaris, and abductor digiti minimi
Trape-zium	Tubercle	• Attachment for flexor retinaculum, opponens pollicis, abductor pollicis brevis, and flexor pollicis brevis • Articulates with scaphoid, 1st and 2nd metacarpals, and trapezoid
Trapezoid	Wedge-shaped	Articulates with scaphoid, 2nd metacarpal, trapezium, and capitate
Capitate	Head	• Attachment for adductor pollicis • Articulates with scaphoid; lunate; 2nd, 3rd, and 4th metacarpals; trapezoid; and hamate • Largest carpal bone
Hamate	Hamulus	Attachment for flexor retinaculum, opponens digiti minimi, flexor carpi ulnaris, flexor digiti minimi; articulates with lunate, 4th and 5th metacarpals, triquetrum, and capitate

(continued)

Bones of the hand *(continued)*

Bone	Characteristic	Significance
Metacarpals (5)	Heads	Articulate with proximal phalanges
Proximal phalanges (5)		Articulate with more distal phalanges
Middle phalanges (5)		
Distal phalanges (4)	Tuberosity	Ungual tuberosity supports the fingernail

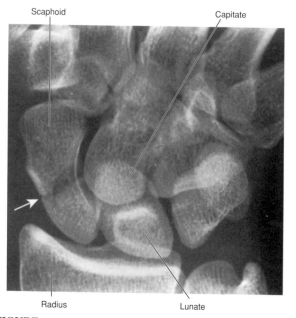

FIGURE 6-4. Scaphoid fracture. The scaphoid is the most frequently fractured carpal bone; fractures may result from a fall on the palm. (From Dudek RW, Louis TM. *High-Yield Gross Anatomy.* 3rd ed. Baltimore: Lippincott Williams & Wilkins; 2008:235.)

Mnemonic

Carpal Bones

She Looks To Pretty, Try To Catch Her
Scaphoid, Lunate, Triquetrum, Pisiform, Trapezium,
    Trapezoid, Capitate, Hamate
The trapezium is nearest the thumb—trapeze-e-thumb.

Clinical Significance

Fractures

The **scaphoid** is the most frequently fractured carpal bone and occurs from a fall on the palm when the wrist is abducted.

Fracture of the 5th **metacarpal**, a boxer's fracture, occurs when an unskilled person punches someone, causing the head of the bone to rotate over the distal shaft.

Injuries of the **phalanges** are common and are extremely painful, often resulting from crush injuries.

Muscles of the hand

Muscle	Proximal Attachment	Distal Attachment	Innervation	Main Actions
Thenar Muscles				
Opponens pollicis	Flexor retinaculum, trapezium	1st meta-carpal	Recurrent branch of median	Rotates and draws 1st meta-carpal medially
Abductor pollicis	Flexor retinaculum, trapezium, and scaphoid	Proximal phalanx of thumb		Abducts thumb, helps opposition
Flexor pollicis brevis	Flexor retinaculum, and trapezium		• Superficial head—recurrent branch of median • Deep head—deep branch of ulnar	Flexes thumb
Adductor pollicis	• Oblique head—2nd and 3rd meta-carpals, capitate and adjacent carpals		Deep branch of ulnar	Adducts thumb

(continued)

Muscles of the hand *(continued)*

Muscle	Proximal Attachment	Distal Attachment	Innervation	Main Actions
	• Transverse head—3rd metacarpal			
Hypothenar Muscles				
Abductor digiti minimi	Pisiform	Proximal phalanx of 5th digit	Deep branch of ulnar	Abducts 5th digit
Flexor digiti minimi	Flexor retinaculum and hamate			Flexes 5th digit
Opponens digiti minimi		5th meta-carpal		Opposes 5th digit with thumb
Short Muscles—Lumbricals and Interossei				
1st and 2nd lumbricals	Tendons of flexor digitorum profundus	Extensor expansions of digits 2–5	Median	Flex digits at metacarpophalangeal joints and extend at interphalangeal joints
3rd and 4th lumbricals			Deep branch of ulnar	
Palmar interossei	2nd, 4th, and 5th metacarpals	Proximal phalanges and extensor expansions of 2nd, 4th, and 5th digits		• Adduct 2nd, 4th, and 5th digits • Flex digits at metacarpophalangeal joints and extend at interphalangeal joints
Dorsal interossei	Metacarpals	Proximal phalanges and extensor expansions of 2nd–4th digits		Abduct 2nd–4th digits; flex digits at metacarpophalangeal joints and extend at interphalangeal joints

Mnemonics

Innervation of Hand Musculature

Meat **LOAF** muscles—Median nerve innervates the first two **L**umbricals, **O**pponens Pollicis, **A**bductor Pollicis Brevis and **F**lexor Pollicis Brevis in the hand.

Interossei Function

PAd and **DAb**—**P**almer interossei **Ad**duct, **D**orsal interossei **Ab**duct.

Hand nerves

Nerve	Origin	Structures Innervated
Median	Union of lateral root (lateral cord) and medial root (medial cord)	Opponens pollicis, abductor pollicis brevis, superficial head of flexor pollicis brevis, and 1st and 2nd lumbricals
Palmar cutaneous branch of median	Median	Sensory over palm, sides of digits 1–3, lateral side of 4th digit, and dorsum of of distal aspect of digits 1–4
Ulnar	Medial cord of brachial plexus	Opponens digiti minimi, flexor digiti minimi brevis, abductor digiti minimi, 3rd and 4th lumbricals, adductor pollicis, deep head of flexor pollicis brevis, and the palmar and dorsal interossei
Palmar cutaneous branch of ulnar	Ulnar	Sensory to medial aspect of palm, 5th digit and medial half of 4th digit
Dorsal cutaneous branch of ulnar		Sensory to medial aspect of dorsum, 5th digit and medial half of 4th digit
Superficial branch of radial	Radial	Sensory to lateral ⅔ of dorsum of hand, thumb and lateral 1½ digits

Vessels of the hand
(Figure 6-2)

Artery	Origin	Description
Superficial palmar arch	Continuation of the ulnar with contribution from radial	Common palmar digital arteries
Deep palmar arch	Continuation of the radial with contribution from the ulnar	Palmar metacarpal arteries

(continued)

Vessels of the hand *(continued)*

Artery	Origin	Description
Common palmar digitals	Superficial palmar arch	Proper palmar digitals
Proper palmar digitals	Common palmar digitals	Supplies digits
Princeps pollicis	Radial	Supplies thumb
Radialis indicis		Supplies 2nd digit
Dorsal carpal arch	Radial and ulnar	Supplies wrist
Palmar carpal arch		

Additional Concept

Venous Drainage

Venous drainage generally parallels arterial supply.

Palmar Arches

The superficial palmar arch is more distal (in line with the distal margin of the extended thumb); the deep arch is more proximal.

Clinical Significance

Palmar Arch

Bleeding is usually profuse and difficult to control when the palmar arches are lacerated. Often, it is necessary to compress the brachial artery in the arm to limit the bleeding.

MISCELLANEOUS

Areas of the upper limb

Area	Structure	Significance
Axilla	4-sided, fat-filled, pyramidal space inferior to glenohumeral joint and superior to axillary fascia: • Apex: cervicoaxillary canal—passageway between neck and axilla • Base: axillary fascia • Anterior wall: pectoralis major and minor	• Permits passage of neurovascular elements to and from the upper limb—contains axillary artery and vein, major portion of the brachial plexus, and lymph nodes

(continued)

Areas of the upper limb *(continued)*

Area	Structure	Significance
	• Posterior wall: subscapularis, teres major, and latissimus dorsi • Medial wall: thoracic wall and serratus anterior • Lateral wall: humerus	• Axillary sheath: extension of cervical (prevertebral) fascia that ensheaths proximal end of neurovascular elements
Quadrangular space	Boundaries: • Superior: teres minor • Inferior: teres major • Medial: long head of triceps brachii • Lateral: humerus	Permits passage of the axillary nerve and posterior humeral circumflex artery to posterior aspect of shoulder
Upper triangular space	Boundaries: • Superior: teres minor • Inferior: teres major • Lateral: long head of triceps brachii	Permits passage of the circumflex scapular artery to posterior aspect of shoulder
Lower triangular space	Boundaries: • Superior: teres major • Medial: long head of triceps brachii • Lateral: medial head of triceps brachii	Permits passage of radial nerve and deep brachial artery to posterior aspect of arm
Cubital fossa	Triangular depression on anterior aspect of elbow, boundaries: • Superior: imaginary line between the medial and lateral epicondyles • Medial: pronator teres • Lateral: brachioradialis • Floor: brachialis • Roof: bicipital aponeurosis	• Contains: brachial artery and its division into radial and ulnar arteries (and their accompanying deep veins), biceps brachii tendon, and median nerve • Median cubital vein lies superficial to bicipital aponeurosis
Carpal tunnel	Cup-shaped (concave anteriorly) passageway from the forearm to the hand; boundaries: • Lateral: scaphoid and trapezoid • Medial: hamate and pisiform • Roof (anterior): flexor retinaculum	Conveys the tendons of the flexor digitorum superficialis, flexor digitorum profundus and flexor pollicis longus, and the median nerve
Deltopectoral triangle	• Triangular area bounded by the clavicle, deltoid and pectoralis major • Covered by clavipectoral fascia	Pierced by cephalic vein, branches of the thoracoacromial trunk and lateral pectoral nerve located within
Anatomic snuff-box	Triangular area bounded medially by the tendon of extensor pollicis longus, laterally by the tendons of extensor pollicis brevis and abductor pollicis longus	• Floor is formed primarily by the scaphoid • Radial artery passes through—the radial pulse may be taken here

Mnemonic

Structures in the Cubital Fossa

TAN—structures found within the cubital fossa from lateral to medial:

Tendon: biceps brachii
Artery: brachial
Nerve: median

Clinical Significance

Axilla

Wounds in the axilla often involve the axillary vein, because of its large size and superficial position.

Carpal Tunnel

Carpal tunnel syndrome results from anything that limits the space in the carpal tunnel and is characterized by loss of sensation over the first digit, the inability to oppose the thumb, and thenar wasting from the compromised function of the median nerve.

Superficial structures of the upper limb

Structure	Course/Significance
Vessel	
Cephalic vein	• Origin: dorsal venous network; runs along lateral aspect of upper limb • Enters deltopectoral triangle, pierces costocoracoid membrane to join axillary vein
Basilic vein	• Origin: dorsal venous network; runs along medial aspect of upper limb • Pierces the brachial fascia at mid-arm to join with the brachial veins to form the axillary vein
Median cubital vein	• Joins the cephalic and basilic veins over the cubital fossa • Supported by the bicipital aponeurosis
Median vein of the forearm	• Origin: dorsal venous network • Courses between and enters the cephalic or basilic veins at the elbow
Dorsal venous network	Highly variable superficial venous network on dorsum of hand
Lymphatics of upper limb	• Superficial lymphatic vessels accompany veins to enter superficial lymph nodes • Includes: cubital and axillary groups

(continued)

Superficial structures of the upper limb *(continued)*

Structure	Course/Significance
Cutaneous Nerve	
Supraclavicular nerves	• Origin: cervical plexus (C3–C4) • Sensory to skin of shoulder
Posterior cutaneous nerve of the arm	• Origin: Radial nerve • Sensory to skin of posterior aspect of arm
Superior lateral cutaneous nerve of the arm	• Origin: continuation of axillary nerve • Sensory to lateral aspect of arm (proximally)
Inferior lateral cutaneous nerve of the arm	• Origin: radial nerve • Sensory to skin over lateral aspect of arm (distally)
Intercostobrachial	• Origin: 2nd intercostal nerve • Sensory to medial aspect of arm
Medial cutaneous nerve of the arm	• Origin: medial cord • Sensory to medial aspect of arm
Medial cutaneous nerve of the forearm	• Origin: medial cord • Sensory to medial aspect of forearm
Posterior cutaneous nerve of the forearm	• Origin: radial nerve • Sensory to posterior aspect of forearm
Lateral cutaneous nerve of the arm	• Origin: axillary nerve • Sensory to lateral aspect of arm
Lateral cutaneous nerve of the forearm	• Origin: continuation of musculocutaneous • Sensory to the lateral aspect of the forearm
Terminal branches of the median	Sensory over palm, sides of digits 1–3, lateral side of 4th digit, and dorsum of distal aspect of digits 1–4
Terminal branches of the radial	Sensory to lateral ⅔ of dorsum of hand, thumb, and lateral 1½ digits
Terminal branches of the ulnar	Sensory to medial aspect of palm and dorsum, 5th digit, and medial half of 4th digit

Clinical Significance

Median Cubital Vein

The **median cubital vein** is the common vein selected for venipuncture because of its accessibility and superficial relationship to the bicipital aponeurosis, which supplies some protection to the underlying brachial artery.

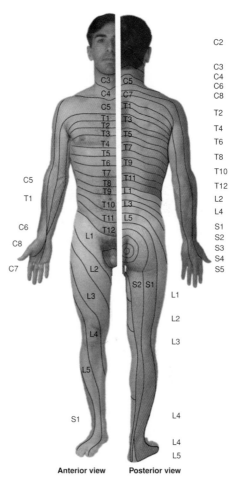

Anterior view   **Posterior view**

FIGURE 6-5. Dermatome maps of the body are based on accumulation of clinical findings following spinal nerve injuries; this map is based on the studies of Keegan and Garrett (1948). Spinal nerve C1 lacks a significant afferent component and does not supply the skin; therefore, no C1 dermatome is depicted. (From Moore KL, Dalley AF. *Clinically Oriented Anatomy.* 5th ed. Baltimore: Lippincott Williams & Wilkins; 2006:53.)

Fascia of the upper limb

Fascia/Connective Tissue	Significance/Structure
Pectoral	Investing fascia of pectoralis major
Axillary	Forms floor of axilla
Clavipectoral	Encloses subclavius and pectoralis minor
Costocoracoid membrane	• Clavipectoral fascia between pectoralis minor and subclavius • Pierced by lateral pectoral nerve
Suspensory ligament of the axilla	• Clavipectoral fascia inferior to pectoralis minor • Supports axillary fascia and forms axillary fossa on abduction
Deltoid fascia	Investing fascia of deltoid is continuous with pectoral and infraspinous fascia
Brachial fascia	• Sheath of deep fascia surrounding arm • Attaches distally to humeral condyles and olecranon process of ulna • Continuous with antebrachial, pectoral, deltoid, axillary, and infraspinous fasciae • Gives rise to medial and lateral intermuscular septa, which divide arm into anterior and posterior compartments
Antebrachial fascia	• Sheath of deep fascia surrounding forearm • Continuous with brachial fascia • Intermuscular septa and the interosseous membrane divide the forearm into anterior and posterior compartments
Extensor retinaculum	Posterior thickening of antebrachial fascia over distal ulna and radius—holds extensor tendons in place
Flexor retinaculum	Anterior thickening of antebrachial fascia over carpal bones—forms carpal tunnel
Palmar fascia	• Continuous with antebrachial fascia • Central portion—palmar aponeurosis
Superficial transverse carpal ligament	Forms base of palmar aponeurosis

Brachial plexus
(Figure 6-6)

Nerve	Significance/Structure
Roots	• Anterior rami of C5–T1 • C5 gives rise to the dorsal scapular nerve and nerve to subclavius • C5–C7 give rise to the long thoracic nerve

(continued)

Brachial plexus (continued)

Nerve	Significance/Structure
Superior trunk	• Formed by the C5 and C6 roots • Gives rise to the nerve to subclavius and the supras-capular nerve
Middle trunk	Continuation of C7 root
Inferior trunk	Formed by the C8 and T1 roots
Divisions	• Each trunk terminates by dividing into an anterior and a posterior division • No branches off the divisions
Lateral cord	• Formed by junction of anterior divisions from the superior and middle trunks • Lateral to axillary artery • Gives rise to the lateral pectoral nerve • Terminates by dividing into the musculocutaneous nerve and lateral root of the median nerve
Posterior cord	• Formed by the posterior divisions of all 3 cords • Posterior to axillary artery • Gives rise to the upper and lower subscapular and thoracodorsal nerves • Terminates by dividing into the axillary and radial nerves
Medial cord	• Formed by the anterior division of the inferior trunk • Medial to axillary artery • Gives rise to the medial pectoral, medial brachial cutaneous, and medial antebrachial cutaneous nerves • Terminates by dividing into the ulnar nerve and the medial root of the median nerve

Mnemonics

Parts of the Brachial Plexus

From proximal to distal:

Real—Roots
Truckers—Trunks
Drink—Divisions
Cold—Cords
Beer—Branches

Terminal Branches of the Brachial Plexus

Terminal branches lateral to medial—

My Audi Races My Uncle.
Musculocutaneous, Axillary, Radial, Median, Ulnar

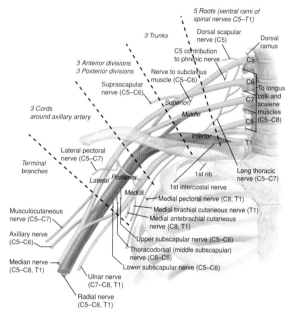

FIGURE 6-6. Brachial plexus. (From Tank PW, Gest TR. *LWW Atlas of Anatomy.* Baltimore: Lippincott Williams & Wilkins; 2009:43.)

Pectoral Nerves

Lateral Less, Medial More—The Lateral pectoral nerve only passes through the pectoralis major, whereas the Medial pectoral nerve passes through both pectoralis major and minor.

Branches of the Posterior Cord

Branches off the posterior cord: **STAR**—**S**ubscapulars (upper and lower), **T**horacodorsal, **A**xillary, **R**adial

Identification Tip

The **musculocutaneous, median,** and **ulnar** nerves form an "M" on the anterior aspect of the **axillary artery**, making their identification a good starting point for the region.

Brachial Plexus Variations

Variations in the form of the **brachial plexus** are common and may include contributions from additional anterior rami such as C4 or T2 or alterations in the **branches, divisions, cords,** or **trunks.**

Clinical Significance

Brachial Plexus Injuries

Injuries to the superior parts of the **brachial plexus** usually result from an excessive increase in the angle between the neck and shoulder, as occurs during a fall increasing the angle between the two or excessive stretching of a baby's head and neck during delivery. Injury to the superior part of the plexus is apparent by the characteristic "waiter's tip" position, in which the limb is medially rotated, the shoulder adducted and the elbow extended.

Injuries to the inferior parts of the brachial plexus occur when the upper limb is pulled superiorly, as in grasping something to break a fall or a baby's upper limb is pulled during delivery. The intrinsic muscles of the hand are involved, resulting in claw hand.

Injury to the Terminal Branches

Musculocutaneous Nerve

Musculocutaneous nerve injury results in paralysis of the muscles in the anterior compartment of the arm and therefore weakening of **elbow** flexion and supination, as well as loss of sensation over the lateral forearm.

Radial Nerve

Injury to the **radial nerve** may result in "wrist drop" as a result of the loss of wrist extensors and the unopposed actions of the flexor muscles.

Median nerve

When the **median nerve** is compromised at the elbow, the 2nd and 3rd digits remain partially extended on attempting to make a fist—the "hand of the benediction."

Ulnar Nerve

The **ulnar nerve** may be compromised as it passes posterior to the **medial epicondyle**, resulting in the characteristic "claw hand," combined with sensory loss over the medial aspect of the palm.

Joints of the upper limb
(Figure 6-3)

Joint	Type	Articulation	Structure	Movements
Sternoclavicular	Synovial	Sternal end of clavicle with manubrium of sternum and 1st costal cartilage	• Anterior, posterior, and interclavicular ligaments strengthen joint • Costoclavicular ligament attaches clavicle to sternum • Divided into 2 compartments by an articular disk	Protraction, retraction, elevation, and depression
Acromioclavicular		Acromial end of clavicle with acromion of scapula	• Coracoacromial and acromioclavicular ligaments strengthen joint superiorly • Coracoclavicular ligament (subdivided into trapezoid and conoid) strengthens joint	Rotation of scapula on clavicle related to movement of the scapulothoracic joint
Glenohumeral (shoulder)		Head of humerus with glenoid fossa of scapula; glenoid fossa deepened by glenoid labrum	• Glenohumeral ligaments strengthen joint anteriorly • Coracohumeral ligament strengthens joint superiorly • Transverse humeral ligament forms	Flexion, extension, abduction, adduction, medial rotation, lateral rotation, and circumduction

(continued)

Joints of the upper limb *(continued)*

Joint	Type	Articulation	Structure	Movements
			canal for tendon of the long head of the biceps brachii • Most joint strength from rotator cuff (supraspinatus, infraspinatus, subscapularis, and teres minor)	
Scapulothoracic	Physiologic joint	Thoracic wall with scapula and associated structures	• No bone to bone articulation • Site of scapula moving on thoracic wall	Elevation, depression, protraction, retraction, and rotation
Humeroulnar and humeroradial (elbow)	Synovial	Trochlea and capitulum of humerus with trochlear notch of the ulna and the head of the radius	Radial and ulnar collateral ligaments strengthen the joint on the lateral and medial aspects	Flexion, extension
Proximal radioulnar joint		Head of radius with radial notch of ulna	Anular ligament of the radius holds the radial head in radial notch of ulna	Supination, pronation by rotation of the radial head
Distal radioulnar joint		Head of ulna with ulnar notch of radius	Anterior and posterior ligaments strengthen joint	Supination, pronation by distal radius rotating around ulnar head

(continued)

Joints of the upper limb *(continued)*

Joint	Type	Articulation	Structure	Movements
Radiocarpal (wrist)		Distal radius with proximal carpal bones	• Anterior and posterior ligaments strengthen joint • Ulnar collateral attaches to styloid process of ulna and triquetrum • Radial collateral attaches styloid of radius and scaphoid	Flexion, extension, abduction, adduction, and circumduction
Intercarpal		Between adjacent carpal bones	Anterior and posterior interosseous ligaments support joint	Gliding, flexion and abduction at midcarpal
Carpometacarpal		Carpals and metacarpals		Flexion, extension, abduction, and adduction
Metacarpophalangeal		Head of metacarpals with proximal phalanges	Palmar ligaments, deep transverse metacarpal, and collateral ligaments support joint	Flexion, extension, abduction, adduction, and circumduction
Interphalangeal		Heads of proximal phalanges articulate with more distal phalanges	Palmar and collateral ligaments support joint	Flexion, extension

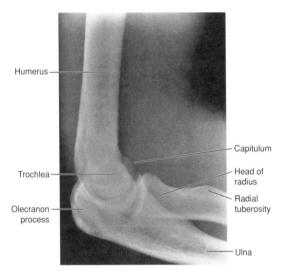

FIGURE 6-7. Lateral elbow radiograph. (From Dudek RW, Louis TM. *High-Yield Gross Anatomy*. 3rd ed. Baltimore: Lippincott Williams & Wilkins; 2008:232.)

Mnemonic

Elbow Movements

Three **B**s **B**end the elbow—

Brachialis
Biceps brachii
Brachioradialis

Clinical Significance

Dislocations

Dislocation of the **acromioclavicular joint**—a shoulder separation, is relatively common in sports or falls that impact the shoulder.

Most dislocations of the **glenohumeral joint** occur inferiorly because of the strong ligamentous and muscular support elsewhere.

Subluxation and dislocation of the head of the **radius**— also known as "nursemaid's elbow" or "pulled elbow"—is common in children that are suddenly lifted by the upper limb.

▍ INTRODUCTION

The head is that portion of the body that sits on the neck; the skeleton of the head is the cranium (skull), which contains the brain and meninges.

CRANIUM

Cranial bone summary
The cranium is divided into a neurocranium and a viscerocranium.

Neurocranium
- encases the brain
- roof—calvarium; floor—cranial base
- formed of bones: frontal, ethmoid, sphenoid, occipital, temporal (2), and parietal (2)

Viscerocranium
- skeleton of the face
- formed of 15 bones: mandible, maxilla (2), inferior nasal concha (2), nasal (2), lacrimal (2), vomer, ethmoid, zygomatic (2), and palatine (2)

Bone	Feature	Significance
Zygomatic arch	Prominence of cheekbone	Formed by union of temporal process of zygomatic bone anteriorly and zygomatic process of temporal bone posteriorly
Hard palate	Bony anterior aspect of palate	Formed by the palatine processes of the maxillae—anterior $2/3$, and the horizontal plates of the palatine bones—posterior $1/3$

(continued)

Cranial bone summary *(continued)*

Bone	Feature	Significance
Frontal	Overall	• Forms anterior aspect of neurocranium • Skeleton of forehead • Forms roof of orbit and floor of anterior cranial fossa
	Supraorbital margin	• Anterior superior aspect of orbit • Possesses supraorbital foramen or notch—transmits supraorbital neurovascular elements
Parietal (2)	Overall	Form lateral aspects of neurocranium
	Temporal lines (superior and inferior)	• Proximal attachment for temporalis and its investing fascia • Form superior border of temporal fossa
	Groove for middle meningeal artery	Conveys middle meningeal artery
Occipital	Overall	Forms posterior aspect of neurocranium
	External occipital protuberance	Attachment for ligamentum nuchae
	Nuchal lines (superior and inferior)	Superior—attachment for sternocleidomastoid, trapezius, and splenius capitis
	Hypoglossal canal	Transmits CN XII
	Jugular foramen	Shared foramen between occipital and temporal bones that transmits CN IX, X, and XI, and internal jugular vein and inferior petrosal sinus
	Foramen magnum	• Site of transition from medulla to spinal cord • Conveys CN XI and vertebral arteries into cranial vault
	Groove for transverse sinus	Location of transverse sinuses
	Internal occipital protuberance	Location of the confluens of the sinuses
	Pharyngeal tubercle	Attachment for pharyngeal raphe
	Occipital condyles	Articulation with atlas
Ethmoid	Cribriform plate	• Forms roof of nasal cavity • Transmits filia olfactoria—CN I
	Perpendicular plate	Forms superior aspect of nasal septum
	Nasal conchae (superior and middle)	• Form superior aspect of lateral walls of nasal cavity • Act as turbinates for inspired air
	Crista galli	Attachment for falx cerebri
Sphenoid	Lesser wing	Forms superior border of superior orbital fissure

(continued)

Cranial bone summary *(continued)*

Bone	Feature	Significance
	Greater wing	Forms inferior border of superior orbital fissure
	Foramen ovale	Conveys mandibular and lesser petrosal nerves
	Foramen rotundum	Conveys maxillary nerve
	Foramen spinosum	Conveys middle meningeal artery
	Sphenopalatine foramen	Conveys sphenopalatine artery and nasopalatine nerve to nasal cavity
	Medial pterygoid plate	Possesses **hamulus** that tensor palati wraps around on way to soft palate
	Lateral pterygoid plate	Attachment for medial and lateral pterygoid muscles
	Optic canal	Conveys CN II and ophthalmic artery
	Sphenoid sinus	Paranasal air sinus that empties into spheno-ethmoidal recess
	Sella turcica	• Forms **hypophyseal fossa**—location of hypophysis • **Anterior and posterior clinoid processes** serve as attachments for diaphragma sella and border the sella turcica, the **dorsum sellae** forms the posterior border of the hypophyseal fossa
	Superior orbital fissure	• Space between lesser and greater wings of the sphenoid • Conveys CN III, IV, and VI, the ophthalmic nerve, and superior ophthalmic vein
	Inferior orbital fissure	• Space between maxilla and greater wing of sphenoid • Conveys infraorbital nerve
Maxilla	Zygomatic process	Articulates with zygomatic bone to form anterior part of cheek
	Infraorbital foramen	Conveys infraorbital neurovascular elements to face
	Alveolar processes	Form sockets for maxillary teeth
	Infraorbital groove	Conveys infraorbital neurovascular elements through orbit
	Incisive canal	Conveys septal branches of sphenopalatine artery and branches of the nasopalatine nerve
	Palatine process	Forms anterior ⅔ of bony palate
	Nasal surface	Forms anterior aspect of lateral wall of nasal cavity
Mandible	Condylar process	• Possesses a **head** and **neck** • Head articulates with temporal bone at temporomandibular joint

(continued)

Cranial bone summary (continued)

Bone	Feature	Significance
	Coronoid process	Distal attachment for temporalis
	Mandibular foramen	• Point along interior of ramus where inferior alveolar neurovascular elements enter mandible • **Lingula** borders entrance, serves as attachment point for **sphenomandibular ligament**
	Mental foramen	Conveys mental neurovascular elements to chin region
	Alveolar processes	Form sockets for mandibular teeth
	Mental spines (superior and inferior)	• Superior—proximal attachment for genioglossus • Inferior—proximal attachment for geniohyoid
	Mylohyoid line	Proximal attachment for mylohyoid
	Ramus	Vertical part between body (angle) and coronoid and condylar processes
	Angle	Bend between ramus and body
	Body	• Horizontal part, forms base of mandible • Possesses alveolar processes
	Mandibular notch	Notch between condylar and coronoid processes
	Mental protuberance	Anterior prominence that forms the chin
Temporal (2)	Squamous part	Flat, lateral aspect; forms part of neurocranium
	Petrous part	• Thick, strong internal part • Houses vestibulocochlear apparatus
	Groove for superior petrosal sinus	Location of superior petrosal sinus
	Groove for sigmoid sinus	Location of sigmoid sinus
	Hiatus for greater petrosal nerve	Conveys greater petrosal nerve into cranial vault
	Hiatus for lesser petrosal nerve	Conveys lesser petrosal nerve into cranial vault
	Internal acoustic meatus	Conveys CN VII and VII from cranial vault into petrous part of temporal bone
	External acoustic meatus	• Bony part of external ear • Conveys sound to tympanic membrane
	Zygomatic process	Articulates with temporal process of zygomatic bone to form **zygomatic arch**

(continued)

Cranial bone summary *(continued)*

Bone	Feature	Significance
	Mandibular fossa	Articulates with head of condylar process of mandible to form temporomandibular joint
	Articular tubercle	Bony prominence anterior to mandibular fossa that forms part of temporomandibular joint
	Styloid process	Proximal attachment for stylohyoid, stylopharyngeus, and styloglossus muscles and for stylohyoid and stylomandibular ligaments
	Mastoid process	• Proximal attachment for posterior belly of digastric • Distal attachment for sternocleidomastoid
	Stylomastoid foramen	Exit for CN VII motor fibers from the cranium
	Petrotympanic fissure	Exit for chorda tympani from the cranium
	Carotid canal	Canal conveying the internal carotid artery and its nerve plexus as they enter the cranium
	Tympanic canaliculus	Conveys tympanic nerve into middle ear cavity
	Jugular foramen	Shared foramen between occipital and temporal bones that transmits CN IX, X, and XI, and internal jugular vein and inferior petrosal sinus
Zygomatic (2)	Zygomaticofacial and zygomaticotemporal foramen	Conveys sensory branches of zygomatic nerve to skin of cheek
	Temporal process	Articulates with zygomatic process of temporal bone to form zygomatic arch
Inferior nasal concha (2)	Overall	• Forms inferior aspect of lateral walls of nasal cavity • Acts as turbinate for inspired air
Palatine (2)	Perpendicular plate	Forms posterior part of lateral wall of nasal cavity
	Horizontal plate	Forms posterior ⅓ of hard palate
	Palatine foramina (greater and lesser)	Convey greater and lesser palatine neurovascular elements respectively
Nasal (2)	Overall	Form bridge of nose
Lacrimal (2)		Form part of medial wall of orbit
Vomer		Forms posteroinferior aspect of nasal septum

Clinical Significance

Fractures of the mandible usually occur in pairs, frequently on opposite sides.

The extraction of teeth leads to the resorption of alveolar bone. The mandible shrinks as a result, possibly leaving the mental foramen open and the mental nerves exposed to pain from dentures.

Additional Concept

The cranial base is divided into three fossae for descriptive purposes:

- anterior cranial fossa—anterior to lesser wings of the sphenoid
- middle cranial fossa—between lesser wings of the sphenoid and the petrous ridge of the temporal bone
- posterior cranial fossa—posterior to the petrous ridge of the temporal bone

Scalp

The scalp consists of the skin and fascia covering the bones of the neurocranium. The first three layers form a single unit that move together.

Layer	Description	Significance
Skin	Thin	Laden with hair follicles and sweat glands
Connective tissue	Thick	Dense, highly innervated
Aponeurosis	Connects frontal and occipital bellies of occipitofrontalis	Causes wrinkling of skin of forehead
Loose connective tissue	Loose, with potential spaces	• Allows scalp to move freely • Potential spaces may allow for fluid accumulation
Pericranium	Dense connective tissue	Periosteum of neurocranium

Clinical Significance

Trauma

Scalp wounds that do not lacerate the epicranial aponeurosis tend not to gape, owing to its strength.

Mnemonic

Layers of the Scalp

From superficial to deep, the layers of the scalp are:

Skin
Connective tissue
Aponeurosis
Loose connective tissue
Pericranium

BRAIN

Brain
(Figure 7-1)

The brain is divided into the cerebrum, cerebellum and brainstem.

- surface area is increased by gyri and sulci
- fissures are deep gyri

Structure	Description	Significance
Cerebrum	• Largest part of brain • Formed of 2 cerebral hemispheres and diencephalon • Cerebrum divided into lobes	Lobes: frontal, parietal, temporal, and occipital
Diencephalon	Located between cerebral hemispheres	Divided into thalamus, hypothalamus, epithalamus, and subthalamus
Cerebellum	Formed of 2 cerebellar hemispheres connected by a midline vermis	Connected to pons of the brainstem by cerebellar peduncles
Brainstem	Divided into midbrain, pons, and medulla	• Midbrain—most rostral, gives rise to CN III and IV • Pons—gives rise to CN V, VI, VII, and VIII • Medulla—caudal-most, gives rise to CN IX, X, and XII

Clinical Significance

Concussion and Contusion

Concussion is a loss of consciousness after a head injury. Contusion results when the pia mater is stripped from the surface of the brain, allowing blood to enter the subarachnoid space.

Cranial nerves
(Figures 7-1, 7-3, and 7-7)

Structure	Description	Significance
CN I	Olfactory	Conveys sense of smell from nasal cavity
CN II	Optic	Conveys visual information from retina
CN III	Oculomotor	• Motor to levator palpebrae superioris, superior, medial and inferior rectus, and inferior oblique • Parasympathetic to sphincter pupillae, ciliaris and superior tarsal muscles
CN IV	Trochlear	Motor to superior oblique
CN V	Trigeminal	Three divisions: 1. Ophthalmic (V_1)—sensory to upper ⅓ of face, cornea, and paranasal sinuses 2. Maxillary (V_2)—sensory to middle ⅓ of face, upper teeth, maxillary sinuses, and palate 3. Mandibular (V_3)—sensory to lower ⅓ of face, temporomandibular joint, anterior ⅔ of tongue, lower teeth, and motor to **muscles of mastication,** anterior belly of digastric, mylohyoid, tensor palati, and tensor tympani
CN VI	Abducens	Motor to lateral rectus
CN VII	Facial	• Motor to **muscles of facial expression,** stapedius, stylohyoid, and posterior belly of digastric • Parasympathetic to submandibular, sublingual and lacrimal glands, and to glands of the nasal and oral mucosa • Sensory to external acoustic meatus • Taste from anterior ⅔ of tongue
CN VIII	Vestibulocochlear	• Vestibular division—conveys balance and equilibrium information from inner ear • Cochlear division—conveys auditory information from inner ear
CN IX	Glossopharyngeal	• Motor to stylopharyngeus • Parasympathetic to parotid gland • Sensory to parotid gland, pharynx, carotid body and sinus, and middle ear • Taste and sensation from posterior ⅓ of tongue
CN X	Vagus	• Motor to pharynx, palate (except tensor palati), and superior part of esophagus • Parasympathetic to thorax and abdomen to mid-transverse colon • Taste from palate and epiglottis • Sensory to external acoustic meatus
CN XI	Spinal accessory	Motor to sternocleidomastoid and trapezius
CN XII	Hypoglossal	Motor to muscles of tongue (except palatoglossus)

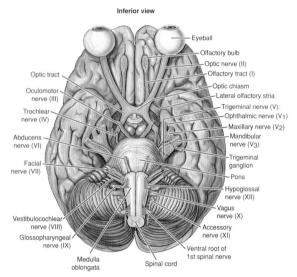

Inferior view

FIGURE 7-1. Cranial nerves, inferior view. (Asset provided by Anatomical Chart Company.)

Clinical Significance

Trigeminal Nerve

Trigeminal neuralgia (tic douloureux) is a sensory disorder of the **trigeminal nerve** of unknown cause. The result is excruciating pain over the face.

Facial Nerve

Injury to the **facial nerve** produces paralysis of the facial musculature (Bell's palsy) on the ipsilateral side, causing the face to droop.

Meninges

The meninges support and protect the brain and cranial nerve roots. They form the subarachnoid space for cerebrospinal fluid.

From superficial to deep, they are the:

- dura mater
- arachnoid mater
- pia mater

Meninges (continued)

Structure	Description	Significance
Dura mater	Separates into 2 layers: periosteal and meningeal in several areas—forming dural sinuses and dural folds (meningeal layer)	• Tough, fibrous layer • Separated from cranium by epidural space • Dural sinuses are blood-filled channels between the periosteal and meningeal layers of dura • Meningeal dura is continuous with the dura mater of the spinal cord
Epidural space	Potential space between cranium and dura mater	Site of epidural hematoma when trauma causes bleeding into space
Subdural space	• Potential space between the dura and arachnoid mater • Filled with a loosely adhered cell layer	Site of subdural hematoma when trauma causes bleeding into space
Arachnoid mater	Middle meningeal layer	Encloses the subarachnoid space
Arachnoid granulations	Evaginations of arachnoid through the dura into the superior sagittal sinus	Convey cerebrospinal fluid from subarachnoid space into the superior sagittal sinus where it mixes with the venous blood
Subarachnoid space	Between arachnoid mater and pia mater	• Contains cerebrospinal fluid, arachnoid trabeculae, and vessels • Irregular enlargements form cisterns
Arachnoid trabeculae	Connective tissue strands that connect the arachnoid and pia mater	Span the subarachnoid space
Pia mater	• Delicate inner layer in contact with the surface of the brain • Deep to the subarachnoid space	Invests spinal blood vessels and the roots of the spinal nerves

Clinical Significance

Vascular and Nerve Supply

The dura mater receives its arterial supply primarily from the **middle meningeal artery**; the veins of the dura follow the arterial branches. The dura mater has rich sensory innervation primarily from the branches of CN V.

Headache

Stretching of the dura mater is a common cause of headaches, as it is sensitive to pain.

Dural folds

Dural folds are formed where the dura mater separates into two layers: periosteal and meningeal.

Structure	Feature	Significance
Cerebral falx	• Infolding of meningeal layer of dura mater as it reflects away from periosteal layer	• Lies in longitudinal fissure of brain • Separates cerebral hemispheres • Superior sagittal sinus lies in attached edge, inferior sagittal sinus lies in inferior free edge; attaches to cerebellar tentorium
Cerebellar falx	• Supports and protects the brain • Possess dural sinuses in margins attached to periosteal layer of dura	• Separates cerebellar hemispheres • Occipital sinus lies in attached edge
Cerebellar tentorium		• Forms a roof over the cerebellum, separating it from the occipital lobe of the cerebrum • Divides cranial cavity into supra- and infratentorial compartments • Anteromedial deficiency—tentorial incisure, allows passage of the brainstem • Straight sinus lies in edge attached to cerebral falx
Sellar diaphragm		• Forms roof over hypophysial fossa • Stretches between clinoid processes • Central deficiency—allows infundibulum to pass through • Cavernous and intercavernous sinuses lie at edges

Additional Concept

Dural sinuses

Dural sinuses are found along the attached edge of dural folds, most often between the periosteal and meningeal layers of dura mater.

Sinus	Feature	Significance
Superior sagittal	• Endothelial-lined venous channels in the attached edge of dural folds, between the layers of dura mater	• Lies in superior, attached edge of cerebral falx • Receives CSF from arachnoid granulations • Lateral extensions—lateral lacunae also receive CSF • Conveys contents to confluens of the sinuses

(continued)

Dural sinuses (continued)

Sinus	Feature	Significance
Inferior sagittal	• Receive cerebral veins and convey venous blood and cerebrospinal fluid (CSF) to the internal jugular vein	• Lies in the inferior, free edge of cerebral falx • Conveys contents to straight sinus
Straight		• Formed by union of inferior sagittal sinus and great cerebral vein • Found in the attachment between the cerebral falx and cerebellar tentorium
Confluence		• Receives blood from straight and superior sagittal sinuses, conveys blood to transverse sinuses • Located near the internal occipital protuberance
Transverse		Pass laterally from confluence of sinus, convey blood to sigmoid sinuses
Sigmoid		• Continuation of transverse sinuses • Continuous with internal jugular vein at jugular foramen
Petrosal (superior and inferior)		• Both drain cavernous sinus • Superior—located in anterolateral attached edge of cerebellar tentorium, drains to junction of transverse and sigmoid sinuses • Inferior—drains into internal jugular vein
Occipital		• Located in attached edge of cerebellar tentorium • Drains blood to the confluence of the sinuses
Cavernous		• Located on either side of the sella turcica, associated with the sellar diaphragm • Communicates with ophthalmic veins and pterygoid plexus • Drains posteriorly via petrosal veins • Walls of sinus contain V_1, V_2, CN III and IV, sinus itself contains internal carotid artery and CN VI • Right and left sinuses connected anteriorly and posteriorly via intercavernous sinuses

Clinical Significance

Cavernous Sinus

Fractures of the cranial base may tear the internal carotid artery as it passes through the cavernous sinus, first causing compression of CN VI and subsequently the structures in the wall of the sinus.

Ventricular system of the brain

The ventricular system of the brain is both the source and pathway for the flow of cerebrospinal fluid (CSF). CSF acts as a buffer, waste depository, and shock absorber for the brain.

Structure	Description	Significance
Lateral (1st and 2nd) ventricles	Cerebrospinal (CSF) flows through **interventricular foramina** into 3rd ventricle	• CSF is created by specialized tufts of pia mater—**choroid plexus,** located in each of the 4 ventricles
3rd ventricle	CSF flows through **cerebral aqueduct** into 4th ventricle	• CSF is absorbed into the venous system through **arachnoid granulations**—evaginations of arachnoid mater into the superior sagittal sinus
4th ventricle	CSF flows through a **median** and 2 **lateral apertures** to enter subarachnoid space	
Subarachnoid space	CSF-filled space between the arachnoid and pia mater	• Surrounds brain • Distended in areas to form **subarachnoid cisterns** (e.g., cerebellomedullary cistern (cisterna magna)—between the medulla and cerebellum

Clinical Significance

CSF may be obtained for diagnostic purposes by a lumbar puncture, or in the case of an infant from the cerebellomedullary cistern via a cistern puncture. Excessive cerebrospinal fluid dilates the brain ventricles (hydrocephalus) and may cause thinning of the cerebral cortex and separation of the bones of the calvaria in infants.

Vasculature of the brain
(Figure 7-2)

Vessel	Origin/Termination	Supplies/Gives Rise To
Arteries		
Internal carotid (2)	Origin: common carotid; enter skull through carotid	• Give rise to ophthalmic, anterior, and middle cerebrals

(continued)

Vasculature of the brain (continued)

Vessel	Origin/Termination	Supplies/Gives Rise To
	canal, and pass through cavernous sinus	• Primary supply to brain
Vertebral (2)	Origin: subclavian; pass through transverse foramina of cervical vertebrae and foramen magnum to enter skull	• Give rise to basilar, posterior inferior cerebellar, and anterior spinal arteries • Supply meninges, brain stem, and cerebellum
Anterior cerebral	Internal carotid	Supply medial aspect of cerebral hemispheres
Middle cerebral		Supply lateral aspect of cerebral hemispheres
Posterior cerebral	Basilar	Supply inferior aspect of cerebral hemispheres
Basilar	Vertebral	• Gives rise to anterior inferior cerebellar, labyrinthine, pontine, superior cerebellar, and posterior cerebral arteries • Supply brainstem, cerebellum, and cerebrum
Anterior communicating	Anterior cerebral	Forms part of cerebral arterial circle
Posterior communicating	Posterior cerebral	• Forms part of cerebral arterial circle • Supply cerebral peduncle, internal capsule, and thalamus

Venous drainage is indirect, draining first to the dural sinuses, then to true veins.

Additional Concept

The **cerebral arterial circle (of Willis)**, is located at the base of the brain and is the anastomosis between the vertebrobasilar and internal carotid systems. It is formed by the posterior cerebral, posterior communicating, internal carotid, anterior cerebral, and anterior communicating arteries.

Clinical Significance

Stroke

An artery supplying the brain can result in a stroke, cerebrovascular accident (CVA) and be evidenced by impaired neurologic function. Occlusion can occur by an embolus (clot) blocking arterial flow. Emboli can originate locally or at some distance (the heart).

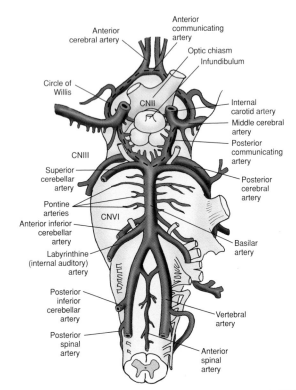

FIGURE 7-2. Circle of Willis. (From Dudek RW, Louis TM. *High-Yield Gross Anatomy.* 3rd ed. Baltimore: Lippincott Williams & Wilkins; 2008:270.)

FACE

Muscles of the face
(Figure 7-3)

Muscle	Proximal Attachment	Distal Attachment	Innervation	Main Actions
Occipito-frontalis—frontal and occipital bellies	Frontal—epicranial aponeurosis Occipital—superior nuchal line	Frontal—skin of forehead Occipital—epicranial aponeurosis	Facial	Elevates eyebrows, wrinkles skin of forehead

(continued)

Muscles of the face (continued)

Muscle	Proximal Attachment	Distal Attachment	Innervation	Main Actions
Orbicularis oculi	Margin of orbit, medial palpebral ligament, and lacrimal bone	Skin around margin of orbit and tarsal plates		Closes palpebral fissure
Corrugator supercilii	Frontal bone	Skin superior to orbit		Wrinkles skin above nose by drawing eyebrows medially
Procerus	Nasal bone and lateral nasal cartilage	Skin of forehead		Wrinkles skin of nose
Nasalis	Maxilla, nasal bone, and lateral nasal cartilage	Alar cartilage, skin of forehead		Flares nostrils, wrinkles skin of nose
Levator labii superioris alaeque nasii	Maxilla	Alar cartilage		Flares nostrils
Orbicularis oris	Maxilla and mandible; skin around mouth	Lips		Closes mouth, protrudes lips
Levator labii superioris	Maxilla	Skin of upper lip		Opens mouth; elevates upper lip
Depressor labii inferioris	Platysma, body of mandible	Skin of lower lip		Opens mouth; depresses angle of mouth
Buccinator	Pterygomandibular raphe; alveolar processes of maxilla and mandible	Angle of mouth		Presses cheek against teeth to keep food out of oral vestibule when chewing
Zygomaticus major	Zygomatic bone			Opens mouth; elevates angle of mouth
Zygomaticus minor		Skin of upper lip		
Levator anguli oris	Infraorbital maxilla	Angle of mouth		

(continued)

Muscles of the face (continued)

Muscle	Proximal Attachment	Distal Attachment	Innervation	Main Actions
Depressor anguli oris	Base of mandible			Opens mouth; depresses angle of mouth
Risorius	Fascia of parotid gland and skin of cheek			Opens mouth
Platysma	Skin of supra-clavicular region	Mandible, skin of cheek and mouth, orbicularis oris		Depresses mandible, tenses skin of neck
Mentalis	Body of mandible	Skin of chin		Elevates skin of chin; elevates and protrudes lower lip

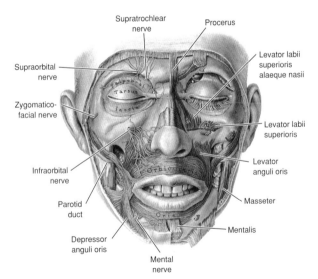

FIGURE 7-3. Anterior view of the face showing the cutaneous branches of the trigeminal nerve, muscles of facial expression, and eyelid (Image from Grant's *Atlas of Anatomy*.)

Vasculature of the face
(Figure 7-4)

Vessel	Origin	Supplies/Gives Rise To
Arteries		
Facial	External carotid	Face
Labial (superior and inferior)	Facial	Lips and nose
Lateral nasal		Nose
Angular		Nose and inferior eyelid
Superficial temporal	External carotid	Lateral aspect of face and temporal region
Transverse facial	Superficial temporal	Face and parotid region
Occipital	External carotid	Back of head
Posterior auricular		Auricle and area posterior to auricle
Mental	Inferior alveolar	Chin
Supraorbital	Ophthalmic	Forehead and scalp
Supratrochlear		
Venous drainage parallels arterial supply.		

Lymphatics of the Head

Lymphatic vessels from the head drain into **deep cervical lymph nodes**, which drain to the **jugular lymphatic trunk**. Collections of lymphatic tissue—tonsils, are found near the opening of the auditory tube—**tubal tonsils**, between the anterior and posterior pillars of the oral cavity—**palatine tonsils**, on the posterior aspect of the tongue—**lingual tonsils** and on the posterior aspect of the nasopharynx—**pharyngeal tonsils**. Together these accumulations of lymphatic tissue form **Waldeyer's Ring**.

Nerves of the face
(Figure 7-3)

Nerve	Origin	Structures Innervated
Sensory		
Branches of the Ophthalmic Nerve		
Supraorbital	Frontal	• Anterolateral scalp and forehead • Frontal sinus • Upper eyelid
Supratrochlear		• Anteromedial scalp and forehead • Upper eyelid

(continued)

Nerves of the face *(continued)*

Nerve	Origin	Structures Innervated
Infratrochlear	Nasociliary	• Medial aspect of both eyelids • Lacrimal sac and caruncle • Lateral aspect of nose
Lacrimal	Ophthalmic	• Conveys parasympathetics to the lacrimal gland • Conjunctiva and skin of upper eyelid
External nasal	Anterior ethmoidal—branch of nasociliary	Majority of nose
Branches of the Maxillary Nerve		
Infraorbital	Maxillary	• Cheek, upper lip, lower eyelid • Maxillary sinus and teeth
Zygomaticofacial	Zygomatic	Cheek
Zygomaticotemporal		Anterior aspect of temporal region
Branches of Mandibular Nerve		
Buccal	Mandibular	• Cheek—skin and mucosa • Buccal gingivae
Mental	Inferior alveolar	• Chin • Mucosa of lower lip
Auriculotemporal	Mandibular—2 roots encircle middle meningeal artery	• Posterior aspect of temporal region • Anterior parts of ear, external auditory meatus and tympanic membrane • Conveys secretomotor fibers to the parotid gland from the otic ganglion
Branches from Cervical Spinal Nerves		
Great auricular	Anterior rami—C2 and C3	• Angle of mandible • Lobe of ear • Parotid sheath
Lesser occipital		Scalp posterior to ear
Greater occipital	Posterior ramus—C2	Scalp of occipital region
3rd occipital	Posterior ramus—C3	Scalp of occipital and suboccipital regions
Motor		
Branches of the facial nerve—temporal, zygomatic, buccal, mandibular, and cervical	Facial (CN VII)	Muscles of facial expression
Mandibular (V_3)	Trigeminal	Muscles of mastication

Additional Concept

Trigeminal Nerve

Branches of the **trigeminal nerve** (CN V) provide most sensory innervation of the face. The three divisions of the trigeminal nerve are the ophthalmic (V_1), maxillary (V_2), and mandibular (V_3) nerves.

TEMPORAL REGION

Temporal region structure

Structure	Description	Significance
Temporal fossa	• Bounded superiorly and posteriorly by superior and inferior temporal lines of the parietal bones • Floor formed by 4 bones that make up the **pterion**	• Proximal attachment of temporalis • 4 bones forming **pterion:** frontal, parietal, temporal, and greater wing of sphenoid
Infratemporal fossa	• Bounded laterally by the zygomatic arch and mandible • Medial border: lateral pterygoid plate • Found posterior to the maxilla	Contains: • Part of temporalis • Medial and lateral pterygoid muscles • Pterygoid plexus of veins • Maxillary artery • Branches of mandibular nerve

Additional Concept

The **temporal region** includes the **temporal**—superior to the zygomatic arch and **infratemporal fossae**—inferior to the zygomatic arch.

Clinical Significance

Mandibular Nerve

A needle is passed through the mandibular notch of the mandible into the infratemporal fossa to anesthetize the mandibular nerve as it emerges from the cranial cavity.

Vasculature of the temporal region

Vessel	Origin	Supplies/Gives Rise To
Arteries		
Maxillary	External carotid	Supplies structures of the temporal region
Deep auricular	Maxillary—1st part	Supplies external auditory meatus
Anterior tympanic		Supplies tympanic membrane
Middle meningeal		Supplies dura mater
Inferior alveolar		• Supplies mandible, floor of mouth, gingivae, and mandibular teeth • Gives rise to **mental**—supplies chin
Deep temporal	Maxillary—2nd part	Supplies temporalis
Muscular (masseteric, buccal and pterygoid branches)		Supply masseter, buccinator and cheek, and the medial and lateral pterygoids
Posterior superior alveolar	Maxillary—3rd part	Supplies posterior maxillary teeth and gingivae
Infraorbital		• Supplies lower eyelid, lacrimal sac, upper lip, and infraorbital region of face • Gives rise to **anterior superior alveolar**—supplies anterior maxillary teeth and gingivae
Descending palatine		Supplies palate and gingivae
Pharyngeal		Supplies superior aspect of pharynx
Sphenopalatine		Supplies lateral nasal wall and septum
Vessel	**Termination**	**Drains**
Veins		
Pterygoid venous plexus	Facial and maxillary veins	Structures in the infratemporal fossa
Venous drainage generally parallels arterial supply in the temporal region.		

Additional Concept

The **maxillary artery** is divided into 3 parts by its relation to the lateral pterygoid muscle.

Nerves of the temporal region

Nerve	Origin	Structures Innervated
Mandibular (V_3)	Trigeminal	• Sensory to structures in the temporal region • Branches convey parasympathetic fibers • Motor to muscles of mastication
Buccal	Mandibular	• Cheek—skin and mucosa • Buccal gingivae
Auriculotemporal		• Posterior aspect of temporal region • Anterior parts of ear, external auditory meatus, and tympanic membrane • Conveys secretomotor fibers to the parotid gland from the otic ganglion
Inferior alveolar		• Forms **inferior dental plexus** that innervates mandibular teeth • Emerges from mental foramen as mental nerve
Lingual		• Anterior ⅔ of tongue and lingual gingivae • Conveys secretomotor fibers to the submandibular ganglion and submandibular and sublingual glands • Conveys special sense of taste from anterior ⅔ of tongue to chorda tympani
Nerve to mylohyoid	Inferior alveolar	Mylohyoid
Chorda tympani	Facial	• Receives taste fibers from anterior ⅔ of tongue from lingual nerve • Conveys presynaptic parasympathetics from CN VII to lingual nerve
Otic ganglion	Innervated by inferior salivatory nucleus	Postsynaptic fibers ride on the auriculotemporal nerve to innervate the parotid gland

PTERYGOPALATINE FOSSA

Pterygopalatine fossa

The pterygopalatine fossa is a small, inverted rain drop shaped fossa, which is positioned for access to multiple areas of the head for distribution of neurovascular elements.

Structure	Description	Significance
Overall	Borders: • Superior—greater wing of sphenoid	Openings and communications: • Superior/anterior—orbit through inferior orbital fissure

(continued)

Pterygopalatine fossa *(continued)*

Structure	Description	Significance
	• Anterior—maxilla • Inferior—pyramidal process of palatine • Medial—perpendicular plate of palatine • Lateral—continuous with infratemporal fossa	• Inferior/posterior—middle cranial fossa through foramen rotundum • Medial—nasal cavity through **sphenopalatine foramen** • Lateral—infratemporal fossa through **pterygomaxillary fissure**
Contents	Maxillary nerve	• Enters fossa via foramen rotundum • Gives off zygomatic nerve in fossa—conveys postsynaptic parasympathetic fibers from pterygopalatine ganglion to lacrimal nerve—to lacrimal gland • Gives off pterygopalatine nerves that suspend ptery-gopalatine ganglion—convey general sense through gang-lion to branches of V_2—supply nasal and oral cavities • Leaves fossa via infraorbital fissure and changes name to infraorbital nerve
	Pterygopalatine ganglion	• Parasympathetic ganglion • Presynaptic innervation is from superior salivatory nucleus via the **greater petrosal nerve**—a branch of CN VII • Greater petrosal joins the **deep petrosal**—sympathetic, to form the **nerve of the ptery-goid canal** • Autonomics leave ganglion to innervate lacrimal, nasal, and oral cavity glands

	Maxillary artery	• Enters fossa via pterygo-maxillary fissure
		• Gives rise to following branches in fossa:
		  1. Posterior superior alveolar
		  2. Descending palatine
		  3. Sphenopalatine
		  4. Infraorbital—gives rise to anterior superior alveolar in infraorbital canal

ORAL REGION

Oral region
(Figure 7-4)

The oral region includes the oral cavity, which extends to the palate superiorly and the palatopharyngeal fold posteriorly, tongue, teeth, and gingivae (gums). The oral cavity receives ingested substances, begins digestion, and forms a bolus that can be swallowed.

Structure	Description	Significance
Oral vestibule	Space between the teeth and gingivae and the lips	• **Oral fissure**—space between upper and lower lips, size varies by orbicularis oris and labial muscles • **Lips**—muscular folds surrounding oral fissure; upper lip sensory by V_2, lower by V_3; **philtrum**—vertical groove in upper lip • **Cheeks**—contain buccinator muscles that function to keep food out of oral vestibule between the occlusal surfaces of teeth
Oral cavity proper	Space contained within superior and inferior **dental arches**—formed of the maxillary and mandibular alveolar processes that contain the teeth	• Continuous posteriorly with the oropharynx • Space occupied by the tongue
Gingivae (gums)	• Mucous membrane covered fibrous tissue • Adherent to alveolar processes and necks of teeth	• Mandibular gingivae innervated by buccal and lingual nerves • Maxillary gingivae innervated by greater palatine, nasopalatine, and superior alveolar nerves—anterior, middle, and posterior
Teeth	• Hard, enamel-covered • Set in alveolar processes of maxilla and mandible • Possess crown, root, and neck • 32 total in adult: 6 molars, 4 premolars, 2 canine, and 4 incisors in each dental arch	• Used in mastication • 20 deciduous teeth in children • Maxillary teeth innervated by superior dental plexus, formed by branches of V_2 • Mandibular teeth innervated by inferior dental plexus, formed by branches of V_3

(continued)

Oral region *(continued)*

Structure	Description	Significance

Tongue	• Muscular organ, mostly contained within oral cavity proper
	• Divided into right and left halves by **midline groove**
	• Possesses:
	  • Root—posterior ⅓
	  • Body—anterior ⅔
	  • Apex—tip
	  • Dorsum—site of lingual papillae: vallate, foliate, filiform and fungiform
	• Inferior surface—has **lingual frenulum**
		• Functions in mastication, deglutition, articulation and taste
		• V-shaped groove on dorsum— **terminal groove** divides tongue into anterior ⅔ and posterior ⅓ parts, center of groove possesses small pit— **foramen cecum** that was the opening of the thyroglossal duct in the embryo
		• Vallate, foliate, and fungiform papillae have taste buds
		• **Lingual frenulum** connects tongue to floor of mouth
		• **Innervation:**
		  • Motor—hypoglossal to all muscles except palatoglossus: pharyngeal plexus
		  • Sensory to anterior ⅔: general sense—lingual, taste—chorda tympani
		  • Posterior ⅓: general sense and taste— glossopharyngeal
		• **Blood supply:** lingual artery, veins parallel arteries

Palate	• Forms roof of oral cavity and floor of nasal cavities
	• Hard palate—bony anterior portion, formed by palatine processes of maxilla and horizontal plates of palatine bones
	• Soft palate—moveable posterior portion of palate; anterior part— composed of **palatine aponeurosis,** posterior part—muscular
		• Hard palate has 3 foramina:
		  1. Incisive fossa: conveys nasopalatine nerve to anterior aspect of hard palate
		  2. Greater palatine foramen: conveys greater palatine vessels and nerves to posterior aspect of hard palate
		  3. Lesser palatine foramen: conveys lesser palatine vessels and nerves to soft palate
		• Soft palate: **uvula** assists in closing oropharynx from nasopharynx during swallowing

Temporo-mandibular joint	• Synovial joint	• Articular disk with anterior and posterior bands divides the joint cavity into 2 separate compartments

(continued)

Oral region *(continued)*

Structure	Description	Significance
	• Between head of mandible with mandibular fossa and articular tubercle of the temporal bone	• Joint supported by a strong **lateral ligament**—a thickening of the joint capsule and by 2 extrinsic ligaments: (1) **stylomandibular ligament** and (2) **sphenomandibular ligament** • Movements: elevation, depression, protrusion, retrusion, and side-to-side grinding movements

Clinical Significance

Temporomandibular Joint

The temporomandibular joint may become arthritic, leading to problems with dental occlusion and joint clicking (crepitus).

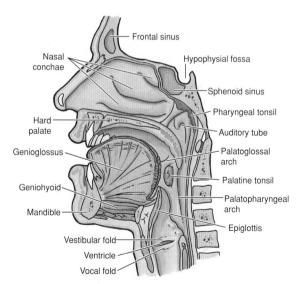

FIGURE 7-4. Nasopharynx, oropharynx, and laryngopharynx. (From Moore KL, Agur AMR. *Essential Clinical Anatomy.* 3rd ed. Baltimore: Lippincott Williams & Wilkins; 2007:621.)

Deep Lingual Veins

The deep lingual veins on the inferior surface of the tongue provide a rapid entry for drugs, such as nitroglycerin for treatment of angina pectoris.

Tongue Tied

An overlarge lingual frenulum (tongue tie) interferes with tongue movement and speech. Frenectomy may be performed to free the tongue.

Salivary glands

There are three pairs of salivary glands:

- parotid
- submandibular
- sublingual

All glands received secretomotor fibers from the parasympathetic nervous system. They function to produce saliva, which binds ingested foot into a bolus and begin the digestive process.

Gland	Description	Significance
Parotid	• Possesses tough fascial sheath—**parotid sheath** • Located anteroinferior to external auditory meatus • **Parotid duct** passes anteriorly to convey secretions into the oral cavity near the 2nd maxillary molar	• Parasympathetic innervation from cells in **otic ganglion** reach target via auriculotemporal nerve • Sympathetic innervation from carotid plexus inhibit secretion • Sensory innervation via auriculotemporal nerve
Submandibular	• Located deep to body of mandible • **Submandibular duct** passes anteriorly to convey secretions into the oral cavity on the surface of **sublingual papilla**—located on either side of the lingual frenulum	• Parasympathetic innervation from cells in the **submandibular ganglion** reach target via the lingual nerve • Sympathetic innervation from carotid plexus inhibit secretion
Sublingual	• Located between the mandible and genioglossus muscle in floor of mouth • Convey secretions into oral cavity via multiple **sublingual ducts**	

Clinical Significance

Sialography

In a sialography, contrast is injected into the submandibular duct to reveal the duct and some of the secretory units of the gland.

Muscles of mastication

Muscle	Proximal Attachment	Distal Attachment	Innervation	Main Actions
Temporalis	Temporal fossa	Coronoid process of mandible	Mandibular	Elevate and retract mandible
Masseter	Zygomatic arch	Lateral aspect of angle and ramus of mandible		Elevate mandible
Medial pterygoid	Medial surface of lateral pterygoid plate	Medial aspect of angle and ramus of mandible		Elevate mandible, produces side-to-side grinding motion
Lateral pterygoid	Lateral surface of lateral pterygoid plate	Disk of temporomandibular joint and condyloid process of mandible		Protrudes mandible, side-to-side grinding motion

Additional Concept

The **masseter** and **medial pterygoid** essentially form a sling attached to the angle of the mandible that elevates the mandible.

Extrinsic muscles of the tongue
(Figure 7-4)

Extrinsic Muscle	Proximal Attachment	Distal Attachment	Innervation	Main Actions
Genioglossus	Superior mental spine of mandible	Dorsum of tongue and hyoid	Hypoglossal	Depresses, protrudes and moves tongue from side to side
Hyoglossus	Hyoid bone	Lateral aspect of tongue		Depresses and retrudes tongue

(continued)

Muscles of the tongue *(continued)*

Extrinsic Muscle	Proximal Attachment	Distal Attachment	Innervation	Main Actions
Styloglossus	Styloid process			Retrudes tongue, elevates sides
Palatoglossus	Palatine aponeurosis	Dorsum of tongue	Pharyngeal plexus	Draws soft palate and tongue together

Additional Concept

The **intrinsic muscles** of the tongue—superior and inferior longitudinal, transverse, and vertical—have no bony attachments and function to alter the shape of the tongue; they are all innervated by the hypoglossal nerve. The extrinsic muscles of the tongue alter the position of the tongue.

Muscles of the palate

Muscle	Proximal Attachment	Distal Attachment	Innervation	Main Actions
Tensor palati	Scaphoid fossa between medial and lateral pterygoid plates	Palatine aponeurosis	Mandibular (V$_3$)	• Tenses soft palate and opens auditory tube during swallowing • Changes direction of pull by wrapping around hamulus of medial pterygoid plate
Levator palati	Cartilage of auditory tube		Pharyngeal plexus	Elevates soft palate
Palatoglossus	Palatine aponeurosis	Tongue		Draws soft palate and tongue together
Palatopharyngeus		Pharynx		Tenses soft palate, elevates pharynx
Musculus uvulae		Uvula		Elevates uvula

Additional Concept

The **palatoglossus** and **palatopharyngeus** are covered by mucosa and are often referred to as the anterior and posterior pillars in dentistry. Between them lies the tonsillar fossa for the **palatine tonsil**.

NOSE AND EAR

Nose
(Figure 7-4)

The nasal apparatus includes the external nose, nasal cavities, and paranasal air sinuses. It functions in olfaction, respiration, filtration and humidification of inspired air.

Structure	Description	Significance

External nose	• Composed of a dorsum (bridge) and apex (tip)
	• **Nares** (nostrils)—are bounded laterally by the alae of the nose and medially separated by the nasal septum; open into the nasal cavities
	• Possesses bony and cartilaginous parts
		• Bony skeleton:
		  • Nasal bones
		  • Frontal bone—nasal part and nasal spine
		  • Nasal septum
		  • Maxillae—frontal process
		• Cartilaginous skeleton:
		  • Lateral cartilages (2)
		  • Alar cartilages (2)
		  • Septal cartilage

Nasal cavities	• Mucosal-lined cavities separated by **nasal septum** • Superior ⅓ is olfactory—contains olfactory receptor cells • Inferior ⅔ is respiratory • Arterial supply: sphenopalatine, ethmoidal (anterior and posterior), greater palatine, superior labial, and branches of the facial arteries • Veins parallel the arteries • Sensory innervation is via nasopalatine, greater palatine, and anterior ethmoidal nerves	• **Nasal septum** composed of: perpendicular plate of ethmoid, vomer, and septal cartilage • **Lateral walls** possess **superior, middle,** and **inferior nasal conchae**—act as turbinates • Spaces inferior to conchae—**superior, middle, and inferior meatuses** • Space superior to superior concha is **sphenoethmoidal recess** • The nasal cavities are continuous with the nasopharynx posteriorly at the **choanae**

(continued)

Nose *(continued)*

Structure	Description	Significance
Paranasal sinuses	Extensions of the nasal cavity into the surrounding bones: • Frontal • Ethmoidal—divided into anterior, middle, and posterior air cells • Sphenoidal • Maxillary	Function as resonant chambers for the voice and in lightening the skull

Clinical Significance

Bloody Nose

Kiesselbach's area is an area on the anterior aspect of the nasal septum where all five arteries supplying the nasal cavity anastomose. It is an area from which may come profuse bleeding.

Deviated Septum

The **nasal septum** is usually deviated to one side or the other, either naturally or as a result of trauma. Deviation can be corrected if it is severe and interferes with breathing or exacerbates snoring.

Additional Concept

The **meatuses** and **sphenoethmoidal recess** are spaces that communicate with sinuses where structures empty into the nasal cavity:

- sphenoethmoidal recess: sphenoid sinus
- superior meatus: posterior ethmoid air cells
- middle meatus: middle ethmoid air cells onto the ethmoid bulla—an expanded ethmoid air cell in the meatus; anterior ethmoid air cell and maxillary sinus into the semilunar hiatus—a depression surrounding the ethmoid bulla; frontal sinus via frontonasal duct into the infundibulum—leads to the semilunar hiatus
- inferior meatus: nasolacrimal duct

Ear
(Figure 7-5)

The ear is divided into external, middle, and inner parts. The external and middle ear transfer sound to the inner ear.

The inner ear contains the organs of hearing and equilibrium.

Part	Description	Significance
External	• Composed of auricle and **external auditory meatus**—bony cartilaginous S-shaped tube • Innervated primarily by auriculotemporal and great auricular nerves • Arterial supply: posterior auricular and superficial temporal arteries • Veins parallel arteries	• Auricle funnels sound into external auditory meatus • External auditory meatus: • Ends at **tympanic membrane** (eardrum)—border between external and middle ear • Filled with hairs and cerumen (wax)
Middle	• Air-filled chamber between the tympanic membrane and inner ear • Connected to nasopharynx by **auditory tube** and mastoid air cells through aditus • Contains **malleus, incus,** and **stapes** • Stapedius and tensor tympani connect to stapes and malleus, respectively • **Chorda tympani** travels through middle ear cavity	• **Auditory tube** equalizes middle ear pressure with atmospheric pressure for optimal hearing • Tympanic membrane vibrations are transferred along the malleus, incus and stapes—the movement of the stapes in the oval window transfers the vibration to the inner ear • Stapedius and tensor tympani dampen sound—innervation: stapedius—CN VII, tensor tympani—CN V
Inner	• Spiraling series of perilymph-containing channels through the petrous part of temporal bone—**bony labyrinth** contains endolymph-filled **membranous labyrinth** • Organs of membranous labyrinth: saccule, utricle, semicircular canals (3), and cochlea • Cochlea is innervated by the cochlear division of CN VIII • Saccule, utricle, and semicircular canals are innervated by the vestibular division of CN VIII	• **Saccule** and **utricle:** located in vestibule of bony labyrinth; contain **macula**—receptor organ that responds to changes in head position • **Semicircular canals:** 3 on each side, contain **crista ampullari**—receptor organs that respond to head acceleration • **Cochlea:** transduces vibrations of stapes in oval window to excitation of CN VIII using **organ of Corti**—receptor organ of membranous labyrinth for hearing

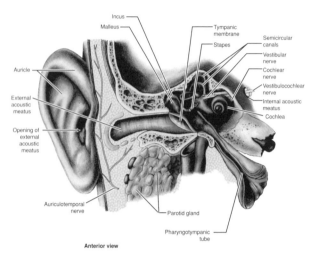

Anterior view

FIGURE 7-5. Anatomy of ear. (From Dudek RW, Louis TM. *High-Yield Gross Anatomy.* 3rd ed. Baltimore: Lippincott Williams & Wilkins; 2008:302.)

Clinical Significance

Ear Infection

Otitis media, an infection of the middle ear cavity, can be secondary to an upper respiratory tract infection. The bulging, red tympanic membrane may perforate as a result of pressure from infection or trauma.

ORBIT

Orbit structure
(Figures 7-3 and 7-6)

The orbits are a pair of bony, pyramidal-shaped cavities in the face that contain:

■ eye
■ extraocular muscles
■ lacrimal apparatus
■ neurovascular elements

Orbit structure *(continued)*

Structure	Description	Significance
Orbit	Bony walls: • Superior—orbital part of frontal and lesser wing of sphenoid • Inferior—maxilla and zygomatic and palatine • Medial—ethmoid and frontal, lacrimal and sphenoid • Lateral—frontal process of zygomatic and greater wing of sphenoid Apex: optic canal Base: orbital margin	• Superior wall contains fossa for lacrimal gland • Medial wall contains lacrimal groove and fossa for lacrimal sac • Inferior wall is separated from lateral by inferior orbital fissure, which conveys the continuation of the maxillary nerve • Optic canal conveys the optic nerve (CN II)
Palpebrae (eyelids)	• Outer surface—thin skin • Inner surface—palpebral conjunctiva • Middle—orbicularis oculi and **tarsal plates:** superior and inferior and **tarsal glands** • **Medial** and **lateral palpebral ligaments** attach tarsal plates to orbit • Eyelashes and ciliary glands • **Lacrimal puncta** open on summit of **lacrimal papilla** on the upper and lower eyelids • **Orbital septum**—an extension of periosteum that connects to the tarsal plates	• Overall: the eyelids protect and moisten the eye, sweeping lacrimal secretions inferomedially toward medial canthus of eye • **Tarsal plates** strengthen eyelids and act as skeleton; the superior tarsal muscle attaches to superior tarsal plate • **Tarsal glands** associated with tarsal plates secrete lipids to prevent eyelids from sticking together and leaking of lacrimal fluid • **Palpebral ligaments** provide attachment for orbicularis oculi • **Orbital septum** helps stop the spread of infection and maintains the orbital fat in place
Eye	• 3 layers of eyeball: 1. Outer—fibrous: sclera and cornea 2. Middle—vascular: choroid, ciliary body composed of ciliaris and ciliary processes and iris that contains dilator pupillae and sphincter pupillae	• Outer layer: **sclera**—white, opaque posterior ⅚, fibrous skeleton of eye; **cornea**—anterior ⅙, transparent, avascular part of refractive media • Middle layer: **choroid**—contains blood vessels; **ciliary body**—contraction of ciliaris by CN III parasympathetics produces accommodation, **ciliary processes** secrete

(continued)

Orbit structure *(continued)*

Structure	Description	Significance

	3. Inner—retina: divided into outer pigmented layer and inner neural layer
	• Spaces within eyeball divided into 3 parts:
	  1. Anterior chamber—between cornea and iris
	  2. Posterior chamber—between iris and lens
	  3. Vitreous body—fills area posterior to lens
	• Lens—flexible avascular part of refractive media of eye; surrounded by lens capsule that is tensed by suspensory ligaments
		aqueous humor and via suspensory ligaments hold the lens; **iris**—continually varies in size to alter size of pupil, dilator under sympathetic control, and sphincter under parasympathetic control (CN III)
		• Inner layer: retina inner neural layer contains photoreceptors and the ganglion cells that form CN II, ends anteriorly at **ora serrata;** area of highest visual acuity—**macula lutea** the center of which has a small pit—**fovea centralis,** located at the center of the visual axis; **optic disk** is a blind spot medial to macula lutea where CN II leaves the eye and the central artery of the retina enters

Lacrimal apparatus	• **Lacrimal glands**—located in the fossa for the lacrimal gland • **Lacrimal ducts**—empty into superior fornix • **Lacrimal canaliculi** convey tears to the **lacrimal sac** via capillary action	• **Lacrimal glands**—produce lacrimal secretions (tears); secretomotor from facial nerve parasympathetics, sympathetics inhibit production • **Lacrimal ducts**—convey lacrimal secretions to conjunctival sac • **Lacrimal sac** is the dilated proximal end of the **nasolacrimal duct** that conveys lacrimal secretions to the inferior nasal meatus

Additional Concept

Conjunctiva

The conjunctiva is a mucous membrane that is loosely adherent to the sclera, known as **bulbar conjunctiva**, where it is invested with blood vessels and on the inner surface of the eyelids as **palpebral conjunctiva**. At the **medial canthus** of the eye—the junction of the upper and lower eyelids on the medial side, the remnant of a human nictitating membrane is evident as a semilunar fold of conjunctiva. The semilunar fold lines the **lacrimal lake**, at the center of which is an elevation, the **lacrimal caruncle** that functions

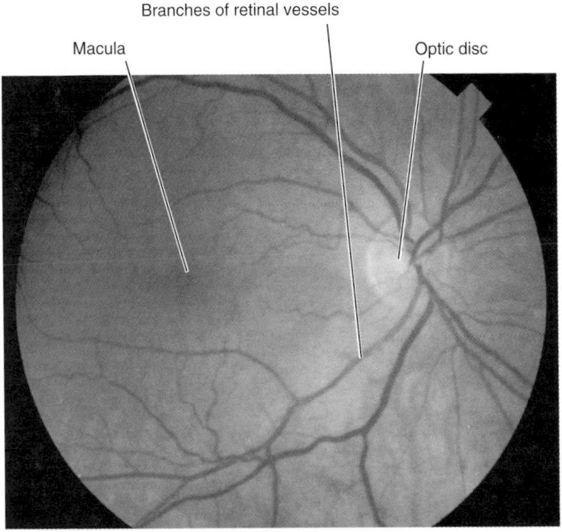

Macula

Branches of retinal vessels

Optic disc

FIGURE 7-6. Retina. (From Dudek RW, Louis TM. *High-Yield Gross Anatomy.* 3rd ed. Baltimore: Lippincott Williams & Wilkins; 2008:298.)

to push the lacrimal secretions to the edge of the lake so that they can be removed by **lacrimal canaliculi.** The lines of reflection between bulbar and palpebral conjunctiva are the **superior** and **inferior fornices.** The conjunctiva line a sac, the **conjunctival sac** the opening of which is the **palpebral fissure**—the space between the upper and lower eyelids. It is into this sac that contact lenses are inserted and eyedrops deposited and into the superior fornix of the sac where lacrimal secretions are emptied via **excretory ducts.**

Clinical Significance

Blowout Fracture

A blow to the orbit is most likely to fracture the relatively thin inferior and medial walls, leading to a blowout fracture with the stronger bony margin intact.

Exophthalmos

Tumors within the orbit or deposition of retrobulbar fat (as in Grave's disease) produce exophthalmos or protrusion of the eye.

Conjunctivitis

The conjunctiva is colorless except when its vessels are dilated (bloodshot eyes) or inflamed from infection (conjunctivitis, or pinkeye).

Extraocular muscles
(Figures 7-7 and 7-8)

Muscle	Proximal Attachment	Distal Attachment	Innervation	Main Actions
Levator palpebrae superioris	Lesser wing of sphenoid	Superior tarsal plate, skin of upper eyelid	Oculomotor and sympathetics— superior tarsal muscle	Elevate upper eyelid
Superior rectus	Common tendinous ring	Anterior hemisphere of sclera	Oculomotor	Elevates, adducts, and medially rotates eye
Inferior rectus				Depresses, adducts, and laterally rotates eye
Medial rectus				Adducts eye
Lateral rectus			Abducens	Abducts eye
Superior oblique	Sphenoid	Passes anteriorly through trochlea, changes direction and attaches to posterior hemisphere of sclera	Trochlear	Depresses, abducts, and medially rotates eye
Inferior oblique	Anterior aspect of floor of orbit	Posterior hemisphere of sclera	Oculomotor	Elevates, abducts, and laterally rotates eye

Additional Concept

Superior Tarsal Muscle

The anterior-most fibers of **levator palpebrae superioris** are smooth muscle—the **superior tarsal muscle**. This smooth muscle component is primarily responsible for keeping the upper eyelid raised.

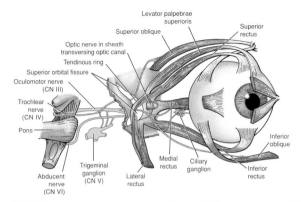

FIGURE 7-7. Innervation of muscles of eyeball. The oculomotor (CN III), trochlear (CN IV), and abducent (CN VI) nerves are distributed to the muscles of the eyeball. The nerves enter the orbit through the superior orbital fissure. CN IV supplies the superior oblique, CN VI supplies the lateral rectus, and CN III supplies the remaining five muscles. (From Moore KL, Dalley AF. *Clinically Oriented Anatomy.* 5th ed. Baltimore: Lippincott Williams & Wilkins; 2006:970.)

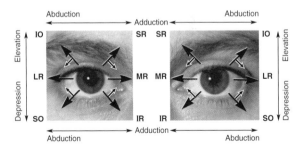

FIGURE 7-8. Eye movements. Large arrows indicate the direction of eye movements caused by the various extraocular muscles. Small arrows indicate either intorsion (medial rotation of the superior pole of the eyeball) or extorsion (lateral rotation of the superior pole of the eyeball). IO = inferior oblique, LR = lateral rectus, SO = superior oblique, MR = medial rectus, IR = inferior rectus. (From Dudek RW, Louis TM. *High-Yield Gross Anatomy.* 3rd ed. Baltimore: Lippincott Williams & Wilkins; 2008:289.)

Clinical Significance

Eye Movements

The medial walls of the orbits are parallel; therefore, the axis of the eye is not in line with the axis of the orbit. The recti muscles attach via a **common tendinous ring** at the apex of the orbit and so produce unwanted movements of the eye when they contract—adduction and rotation. The **superior** and **inferior oblique** muscles offset the rotation and adduction of the eye by the recti to get a more straightforward elevation or depression.

Fascial Sheath of the Eyeball

The eye is surrounded by the **fascial sheath of the eyeball**, which forms a "socket" into which the eyeball sits and that is attached to and pierced by the extraocular muscles. Extensions of the sheath are attached to the orbit as **medial** and **lateral check ligaments** that limit adduction and abduction of the eye. The check ligaments blend with the fascia of the inferior rectus and inferior oblique muscles to form the **suspensory ligament of the eyeball**, a hammock-like sling that supports the eye. The fascial sheath of the eyeball forms the socket into which a prosthetic eye is inserted, still allowing for relatively natural movement because of the connection to the extraocular muscles.

Mnemonic

To recall the innervation pattern of the extraocular muscles use this "formula":

$[SO_4LR_6]_3$ Superior Oblique by CN IV; Lateral Rectus by CN VI and all the rest by CN III.

Vasculature of the orbit

Vessel	Origin	Supplies/Gives Rise To
Arteries		
Ophthalmic	Internal carotid	Supplies structures of orbit, face, and scalp
Central artery of the retina	Ophthalmic	Supplies retina
Supraorbital		Supplies forehead and scalp
Supratrochlear		
Dorsal nasal		Supplies nose

(continued)

Vasculature of the orbit *(continued)*

Vessel	Origin	Supplies/Gives Rise To
Lacrimal		Supplies eyelids, conjunctiva, and lacrimal gland
Ethmoidal (anterior and posterior)		Supplies ethmoidal air cells and nasal cavity
Posterior ciliary (short and long)		Supplies middle layer of eye
Anterior ciliary		

Vessel	Termination	Drains
Veins		
Scleral venous sinus	Vorticose vein	Aqueous humor from anterior chamber
Vorticose	Ophthalmic veins	Middle layer of eye
Central vein of the retina	Cavernous sinus or inferior ophthalmic vein	Retina
Superior ophthalmic	Cavernous sinus and the inferior ophthalmic also drains into the pterygoid venous plexus	Eye and orbit
Inferior ophthalmic		

Nerves of the orbit
(Figure 7-7)

Nerve	Origin	Structures Innervated
Frontal	Ophthalmic	Upper eyelid, scalp, and forehead via two terminal branches—supraorbital and supratrochlear
Nasociliary	Ophthalmic	Eye, face, and nasal cavity
Ethmoidal (anterior and posterior)	Nasociliary	Sphenoid and ethmoid air cells and nasal cavity
Long ciliary		• Eye • Conveys sympathetics to iris and sensation from cornea
Short ciliary	Ciliary ganglion	• Eye • Conveys sympathetics and parasympathetics from CN III to iris and ciliaris
Lacrimal	Ophthalmic	• Conveys parasympathetics to the lacrimal gland from V_2 • Conjunctiva and skin of upper eyelid
Ciliary ganglion	Innervated by accessory oculomotor nucleus	• Presynaptic parasympathetics are conveyed via CN III • Postganglionics are conveyed via short ciliary nerves to ciliaris and sphincter pupillae

PARASYMPATHETIC GANGLIA IN THE HEAD

Parasympathetic ganglia in the head

Ganglia	Afferents	Efferents
Ciliary	Accessory oculomotor nucleus via CN III	Postsynaptics innervate sphincter pupillae and ciliaris
Otic	Inferior salivatory nucleus via CN IX	Postsynaptics innervate parotid gland
Pterygopalatine	Superior salivatory nucleus via CN VII branch—greater petrosal nerve	Postsynaptics innervate oral and nasal mucosa and the lacrimal gland
Submandibular	Superior salivatory nucleus via CN VII branch—chorda tympani	Postsynaptics innervate the sublingual and submandibular glands

Mnemonic

The acronym C-O-P-S is a useful way to remember the four parasympathetic ganglia of the head.

INTRODUCTION

The neck supports the head and connects it to the trunk. It not only houses organs of its own, but serves as a passageway for structures coursing between the head and trunk.

NECK

Skeleton of the Neck

The skeleton of the neck consists of the seven cervical vertebrae—presented with the back, the sternum—presented with the thorax, the clavicles—presented with the upper limb and the hyoid bone.

The hyoid bone does not articulate with any other bones. It functions primarily as a muscle attachment for muscles of the tongue and larynx.

Clinical Significance

Hyoid Fracture

Fractures of the hyoid are common in persons who are strangled. The result is an inability to elevate the hyoid, which makes swallowing and the prevention of ingested substances from entering the airway difficult.

Fascia and spaces of the neck
(Figure 8-1)

The neck is surrounded by a fatty layer of superficial fascia; the deep fascia of the neck divides it into compartments, facilitates movement, and determines the spread of infection.

Fascia and spaces of the neck (continued)

Structure	Description
Superficial cervical fascia	• Overlies the deep cervical fascia • Contains the platysma • Contains neurovascular, lymphatic, and fat
Deep Cervical Fascia	
Investing	• Surrounds entire neck like a sleeve • Splits to enclose the sternocleidomastoid and trapezius muscles and submandibular and parotid gland—forms fibrous capsule • Continuous with nuchal ligament
Prevertebral	• Encloses the vertebral column, longus coli, scalenes—anterior, middle and posterior, longus capitis, and deep cervical muscles • An extension of prevertebral fascia forms the **axillary sheath**—that surrounds the axillary vessels and brachial plexus
Pretracheal	• Encloses the infrahyoid muscles, thyroid gland, trachea, and esophagus • Continuous with buccopharyngeal fascia
Carotid sheath	• Encloses the common carotid artery, internal jugular vein, and vagus nerve • Composed of contributions from investing, prevertebral and pretracheal fascia
Buccopharyngeal fascia	• Encloses the pharynx • Continuous with pretracheal fascia
Spaces of the Neck	
Retropharyngeal space	• Between prevertebral and buccopharyngeal fascia • Subdivided by alar fascia • Permits movement of the viscera during swallowing • Also called—danger space, because it is a pathway for infection to spread between the neck and posterior mediastinum

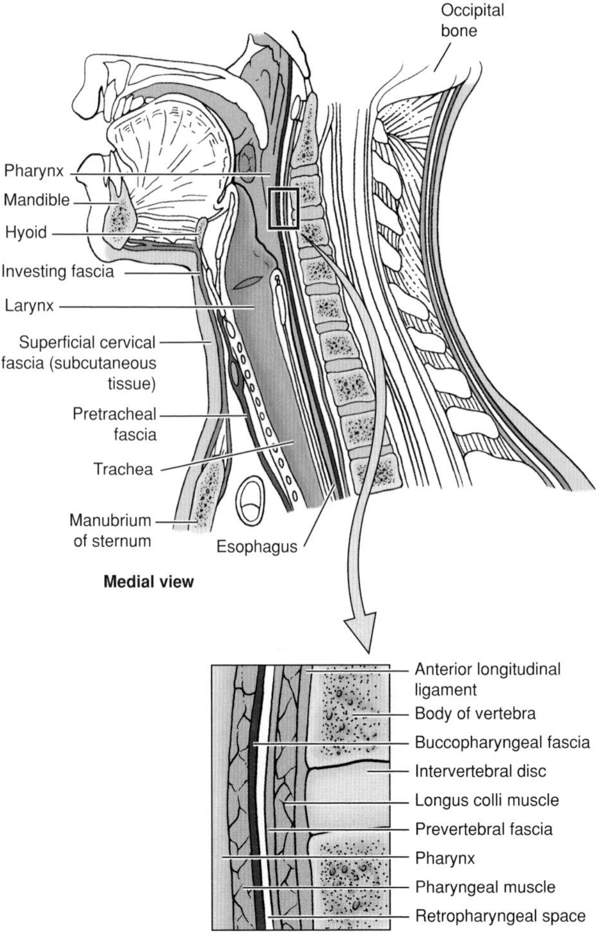
Occipital bone
Pharynx
Mandible
Hyoid
Investing fascia
Larynx
Superficial cervical fascia (subcutaneous tissue)
Pretracheal fascia
Trachea
Manubrium of sternum
Esophagus
Medial view
Anterior longitudinal ligament
Body of vertebra
Buccopharyngeal fascia
Intervertebral disc
Longus colli muscle
Prevertebral fascia
Pharynx
Pharyngeal muscle
Retropharyngeal space

FIGURE 8-1. Sections of head and neck demonstrating cervical fascia. (From Moore KL, Dalley AF. *Clinically Oriented Anatomy.* 5th ed. Baltimore: Lippincott Williams & Wilkins; 2006:1050.)

Regions of the neck
(Figures 8-2, 8-3, and 8-6)

The neck is divided into four regions.

Region	Description and Contents

Anterior cervical (anterior triangle of the neck)	• Borders:
	  • Anterior—midline of neck
	  • Posterior—anterior border of sternocleido-mastoid
	  • Inferior—junction of midline of neck and sternocleidomastoid
	  • Superior—mandible
	  • Roof—investing layer of deep cervical fascia
	  • Floor—pretracheal fascia investing pharynx, larynx, and thyroid
	• Nerves in region:
	  • Transverse cervical—sensory to skin of region
	  • Hypoglossal—supplies tongue
	  • Vagus
	  • Glossopharyngeal
	• Arteries in region:
	  • Common carotid—terminate in region to form internal and external carotid arteries
	  • Internal carotid—no branches in neck; enter cranium via carotid canal
	  • External carotid—terminates as maxillary and superficial temporal arteries; before termination gives:
	    1. Ascending pharyngeal
	    2. Occipital
	    3. Posterior auricular
	    4. Superior thyroid
	    5. Lingual
	    6. Facial
	• Veins in region:
	  • Internal jugular—begins at jugular foramen as continuation of sigmoid sinus, joins subclavian to form brachiocephalic vein, receives—inferior petrosal sinus, facial, lingual, pharyngeal, and thyroid veins—superior and middle
	  • Anterior jugular
	• Subdivided by digastric and omohyoid into:
	  • Submental triangle—unpaired; between anterior bellies of digastrics, mandibular symphysis and hyoid; contains—submental nodes

(continued)

Regions of the neck (continued)

Region	Description and Contents
	• Submandibular triangle—between mandible and anterior and posterior bellies of digastric; contains—submandibular gland and nodes, hypoglossal nerve (CN XII), facial artery, and vein
	• Carotid triangle—between superior belly of omohyoid, posterior belly of digastric, and anterior border of sternocleidomastoid; contains—common carotid artery and branches, vagus, spinal accessory and hypoglossal nerves, cervical plexus, thyroid gland, larynx, pharynx, and cervical nodes
	• Muscular triangle—between superior belly of omohyoid, anterior border of sternocleido-mastoid, and midline of neck; contains—infrahyoid muscles, thyroid, and parathyroid glands

Lateral cervical (posterior triangle of the neck)	• Borders:
	  • Anterior—posterior border of sternocleido-mastoid
	  • Posterior—anterior border of trapezius
	  • Inferior—clavicle
	  • Superior—junction of sternocleidomastoid and trapezius
	  • Roof—investing layer of deep cervical fascia
	  • Floor—prevertebral layer of deep cervical fascia that covers the middle and posterior scalenes, levator scapulae, and splenius capitis
	• Nerves in region:
	  • Spinal accessory (CN XI), supplies sternocleido-mastoid and trapezius
	  • Brachial plexus—roots and trunks, supplies upper limb
	  • Suprascapular nerve—supplies supra- and infraspinatus
	  • Cervical plexus—C1–C4: give rise to phrenic nerve (C3–C5) that supplies the diaphragm, ansa cervicalis that supplies infrahyoid muscles, and cutaneous branches: lesser occipital, great auricular, transverse cervical, and supra-clavicular, emerge from **nerve point of the neck**—a quarter-sized area midway along the posterior border of sternocleidomastoid

(continued)

Regions of the neck *(continued)*

Region	Description and Contents

	• Arteries in region:
	  • Transverse cervical—from thyrocervical trunk
	  • Suprascapular—from thyrocervical trunk
	  • Occipital—from external carotid artery
	  • Subclavian—3rd part, supplies upper limb
	• Veins in the region:
	  • External jugular—formed by junction of retromandibular and posterior auricular veins, terminates in subclavian
	  • Subclavian—drains upper limb, joins internal jugular to form brachiocephalic vein
	• Subdivided by inferior belly of omohyoid into:
	  • Occipital triangle—superior to omohyoid
	  • Omoclavicular triangle—inferior to omohyoid

Posterior cervical	• Located posterior to anterior border of trapezius • Contains trapezius, suboccipital triangle—lies deep

Additional Concept

Subclavian Artery

The subclavian artery passes posterior to the anterior scalene, whereas the vein passes anterior.

Carotid Artery

In the carotid triangle, the common carotid artery divides into internal and external carotid arteries. At the bifurcation is the **carotid sinus**—a dilation of the internal carotid that functions as a baroreceptor—measures blood pressure, innervated by CN IX. The **carotid body** also lies near the bifurcation and functions as a chemoreceptor—measures oxygen levels in blood, it is also innervated by CN IX.

Clinical Significance

External Jugular Vein

The external jugular vein may become prominent and evident throughout its course as a result of increased venous pressure as occurs in heart failure.

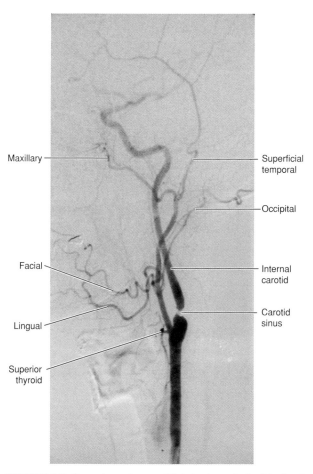

Maxillary

Superficial
temporal

Occipital

Facial

Internal
carotid

Lingual

Carotid
sinus

Superior
thyroid

FIGURE 8-2. Lateral arteriogram (digital subtraction) of the head and neck region with a blocked internal carotid artery. The most common location of atherosclerosis in the carotid artery is at the **bifurcation of the common carotid artery.** Carotid artery plaques are usually ulcerated plaques. (From Dudek RW, Louis TM. *High-Yield Gross Anatomy.* 3rd ed. Baltimore: Lippincott Williams & Wilkins; 2008:268.)

Muscles of the neck
(Figures 8-3 and 8-6)

Muscle	Proximal Attachment	Distal Attachment	Innervation	Main Actions
Sternocleidomastoid	Manubrium and clavicle	Mastoid process and superior nuchal line	Spinal accessory	Laterally flexes and extends neck; rotates head
Suprahyoids—Superior to the Hyoid				
Mylohyoid	Mylohyoid line of mandible	Mylohyoid raphe and hyoid	Nerve to mylohyoid (V_3)	Elevates hyoid
Digastric	Anterior belly—mandible; posterior belly—temporal bone	Intermediate tendon attached to hyoid by connective tissue	Anterior belly—nerve to mylohyoid (V_3); posterior belly—facial	Depresses mandible, elevates hyoid
Geniohyoid	Inferior mental spine of mandible	Hyoid	C1 via hypoglossal	Elevates hyoid
Stylohyoid	Styloid process		Facial	
Infrahyoids—Inferior to the Hyoid				
Omohyoid	Scapula	Hyoid	Ansa cervicalis	Depresses hyoid
Sternothyroid	Sternum	Thyroid cartilage		
Sternohyoid		Hyoid		
Thyrohyoid	Thyroid cartilage		C1 via hypoglossal	
Prevertebral				
Longus coli	C1–C6 vertebrae	C3–T3 vertebrae	Anterior rami of C2–C6	Flexes and rotates neck
Longus capitis	Occipital bone	C3–C6 vertebrae	Anterior rami of C1–C3	Flexes head
Rectus capitis (anterior and lateral)		C1 vertebra	Anterior rami of C1–C2	
Anterior scalene	C4–C6 vertebrae	1st rib	Anterior rami cervical spinal nerves	
Middle scalene				Laterally flexes neck
Posterior scalene		2nd rib		

The trapezius is described with the shoulder region of the upper limb. The platysma is described with the muscles of the face.

Additional Concept

Innervation

The **ansa cervicalis** is a loop in the cervical plexus consisting of fibers from the first three cervical nerves. Fibers from C1–C2 form the superior root, whereas fibers from C2–C3 form the inferior root that unite to form the ansa cervicalis.

Clinical Significance

Torticollis

Torticollis is a contraction of the cervical muscles, most commonly the sternocleidomastoid, which produces a twisting of the neck and slanting of the head.

Root of the neck

The root of the neck is the area of junction between the inferior aspect of the neck and the superior aspect of the thorax.

Feature	Description	Significance

Nerves	• Vagus
	  • Right recurrent laryngeal
	  • Left recurrent laryngeal
	• Phrenic
	• Sympathetic trunks
		• Vagus—located in carotid sheath; right recurrent laryngeal arises after right vagus passes over subclavian artery, left recurrent laryngeal arises after left vagus nerve passes over arch of aorta; recurrent laryngeals ascend in tracheoesophageal groove to supply trachea, esophagus and larynx
		• Phrenic—C3–C5; sensory and motor to diaphragm
		• Sympathetic trunks—3 ganglia: superior, middle, and inferior; postsynaptics conveyed via gray communicating branches to cervical spinal nerves, cardiopulmonary splanchnic nerves to thoracic viscera, and the periarterial plexus to head and neck viscera

Arteries	• Brachiocephalic trunk • Subclavian—right and left	• Brachiocephalic trunk terminates by dividing into right common carotid and right subclavian arteries • Right subclavian is a branch of brachiocephalic trunk; left is a branch of the arch of the aorta
Veins	• External jugular • Anterior jugular • Subclavian	• External jugular drains scalp and face; empties into subclavian

(continued)

Root of the neck (continued)

Feature	Description	Significance
		• Anterior jugular formed by submandibular veins, unites with contralateral counterpart to form the **jugular venous arch** superior to sternum; empties into external jugular • Subclavian vein begins as axillary vein crosses 1st rib; ends by joining internal jugular vein to form brachiocephalic at the **venous angle**—place where thoracic duct and right lymphatic duct typically join venous system on left and right sides respectively

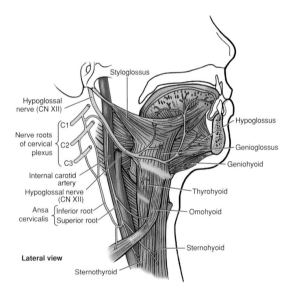

FIGURE 8-3. Distribution of hypoglossal nerve (CN XII). CN XII leaves the cranium through the hypoglossal canal and passes deep to the mandible to enter the tongue, where it supplies all intrinsic and extrinsic lingual muscles, except the palatoglossus. CN XII is joined immediately distal to the hypoglossal canal by a branch conveying fibers from the C1 and C2 loop of the cervical plexus. These fibers hitch a ride with CN XII, leaving it as the superior root of the ansa cervicalis and the nerve to the thyrohyoid muscle. (From Moore KL, Dalley AF. *Clinically Oriented Anatomy.* 5th ed. Baltimore: Lippincott Williams & Wilkins; 2006:1105.)

Additional Concept

Subclavian Arteries

The subclavian arteries are divided into three parts by the anterior scalene muscle. Part 1 is proximal, Part 2 is deep, and Part 3 is distal to the muscle.

Part 1 branches—

- vertebral—runs superiorly in transverse cervical foramina, enters cranium through foramen magnum to supply brain
- internal thoracic—supplies structures in thorax
- thyrocervical—gives rise to inferior thyroid artery: to neck viscera, suprascapular: to scapular region, transverse cervical: to lateral cervical region, and ascending cervical: to neck musculature

Part 2 branches—

- costocervical trunk—gives rise to superior intercostal: to first two intercostal spaces and deep cervical: to neck musculature

Part 3 branches—

- dorsal scapular—supplies rhomboids and levator scapulae and the scapular region

Sympathetic Trunks

The inferior cervical and first thoracic sympathetic ganglia often fuse to form the cervicothoracic or stellate ganglion.

Mnemonic

Phrenic Nerve

Nerve roots in the phrenic nerve: C3, C4, and C5 keep the diaphragm alive.

Clinical Significance

Subclavian Vein

The subclavian vein is a common point of entry for central line placement.

Lymphatics of the neck

Superficial lymphatic drainage of the neck is to superficial cervical lymph nodes located along the external jugular vein. Superficial drainage and drainage from deep structures is conveyed to deep cervical lymph nodes, generally found along the internal jugular vein. Efferents from the deep cervical nodes form the jugular lymphatic trunks that empty lymph into the right lymphatic or thoracic duct.

Structure	Description	Drainage
Thyroid	Lymphatic vessels communicate in a network around the fibrous capsule of the gland	The network of vessels drain to prelaryngeal, pretracheal, and paratracheal nodes, which drain into deep cervical nodes
Parathyroid	Lymphatic vessels drain glands	Parathyroid vessels drain into deep cervical and paratracheal nodes
Larynx	Lymphatic vessels accompany laryngeal arteries	• Vessels superior to vocal folds follow superior laryngeal artery to the deep cervical nodes • Vessels inferior to vocal folds drain into pretracheal or paratracheal nodes, which drain to deep cervical nodes
Pharynx	Lymphatic vessels from the tonsils drain to nodes near the angle of the mandible	The lymph from the tonsils is referred to the **jugulodigastric node**

Additional Concept

Tonsillar Ring

The palatine, lingual, tubal, and pharyngeal tonsils form the **tonsillar ring** (Waldeyer's Ring)—a ring of lymphatic tissue around the superior aspect of the pharynx.

Clinical Significance

Tonsillectomy

Tonsillectomy is performed by removing the palatine tonsil and its fascia from the tonsillar bed. Inflammation of the pharyngeal tonsils is adenoiditis. Inflamed adenoids may interfere with nasal breathing and allow infection to spread to the middle ear cavity through the auditory tube.

ENDOCRINE ORGANS IN THE NECK

Thyroid and parathyroid
(Figures 8-2 and 8-6)

The endocrine organs of the neck include the thyroid and parathyroid glands. The thyroid gland—located in the anterior aspect of the neck, produces thyroid hormone and calcitonin, whereas the four parathyroid glands—embedded in the posterior aspect of the thyroid gland—produce parathyroid hormone.

Gland	Feature	Description
Thyroid	• Lobes—right and left are connected by an isthmus • Arterial supply—superior and inferior thyroid arteries • Venous drainage—superior, middle and inferior thyroid veins • Innervation—sympathetic	• Gland is surrounded by a fibrous capsule and the pretracheal layer of deep cervical fascia • Superior and middle thyroid veins drain into the internal jugular veins, whereas the inferior veins drain the brachiocephalic veins • Sympathetic innervation is from the cervical sympathetic ganglia; the postganglionics follow arteries to the gland and cause vasoconstriction
Parathyroid	• Arterial supply—inferior thyroid glands • Venous drainage—drain into the thyroid veins • Innervation—sympathetic	Sympathetic innervation is from the cervical sympathetic ganglia; the postganglionics follow arteries to the gland and cause vasoconstriction

Additional Concept
Thyroid Ima Artery

The thyroid ima artery is present in approximately 10% of people. It has a variable origin, often from the aorta, and, when present, supplies the trachea and isthmus of the thyroid. This midline artery must be considered during procedures in the midline of the neck.

Clinical Significance
Goiter

Enlargement of the thyroid gland—goiter, results from iodine deficiency. The enlarged gland may compress nearby structures.

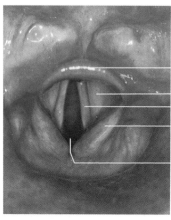

Epiglottis

Vestibular fold

Vocal fold

Aryepiglottic fold

Rima glottidis

FIGURE 8-4. Laryngeal cartilages. Photograph depicting the structures observed during inspection of the vocal cords using a laryngeal mirror. (From Dudek RW, Louis TM. *High-Yield Gross Anatomy.* 3rd ed. Baltimore: Lippincott Williams & Wilkins; 2008:280.)

RESPIRATORY STRUCTURES IN THE NECK

Larynx and trachea
(Figures 8-2, 8-4, and 8-5)

The larynx routes air into the respiratory tract, food into the esophagus, blocks the airway during swallowing, and produces the voice.

The trachea, presented in detail in the thorax chapter (see Chapter 1), extends from the inferior border of the cricoid cartilage of the larynx to its termination in the thorax at the level of the sternal angle as the right and left primary bronchi.

Structure	Description	Significance
Laryngeal inlet	Space bounded by aryepiglottic folds and epiglottis	Entrance into the larynx at which point the vestibule of the larynx is continuous with the laryngopharynx
Laryngeal vestibule	Space bounded by laryngeal inlet superiorly and vestibular folds inferiorly	Space contained between the quadrangular membrane

(continued)

Larynx and trachea *(continued)*

Structure	Description	Significance
Laryngeal ventricle	Lateral extension of laryngeal cavity between vestibular and vocal folds	**Laryngeal saccule**—blind-ended, mucous-secreting pocket that opens into ventricle
Infraglottic cavity	Space bounded by vocal folds superiorly and inferior border of cricoid cartilage inferiorly	Continuous inferiorly with lumen of trachea
Vestibular folds	Mucosa covered folds that project into laryngeal cavity	• Contain vestibular ligament • Space between—**rima vestibuli** • Adducting vestibular folds prevents ingested substances from entering airway
Vocal folds		• Contain vocal ligament and **vocalis:** lateral to vocal ligaments, involved in whispering • Adducting vocal folds prevents ingested subances from entering airway
Glottis	Vocal folds and space between them—**rima glottidis**	Varying the tension and length of the vocal folds varies size of rima glottidis to produce varying pitch for speech

Additional Concept

Blood Supply to the Larynx

The superior laryngeal artery, a branch of the superior thyroid artery, passes through the thyrohyoid membrane with the internal laryngeal nerve to anastomose with the internal laryngeal artery, a branch of the inferior thyroid artery that accompanies the inferior laryngeal nerve. The venous drainage parallels arterial supply.

Clinical Significance

Valsalva Maneuver

In the Valsalva maneuver, the vestibular and vocal folds are tightly adducted after a deep inspiration. Contraction of the abdominal muscles increases intrathoracic and intraabdominal pressures, thereby impeding venous return to the heart.

Skeleton of the larynx
(Figure 8-5)

The skeleton of the larynx consists of nine cartilages that are connected by membranes and ligaments.

Structure	Description	Significance
Thyroid cartilage	Composed of 2 **laminae**— possess a set of **superior** and **inferior horns** on their posterior borders	• The anterior junction of the laminae form the **laryngeal prominence** or Adam's apple • The superior horn and border of the cartilage attach to the hyoid by the **thyrohyoid membrane** • The inferior horns articulate with the cricoid cartilage at the **cricothyroid joint**
Cricoid cartilage	Complete cartilaginous ring inferior to thyroid cartilage	• Connected to thyroid cartilage by **median cricothyroid ligament** • Connected to 1st tracheal ring by **cricotracheal ligament**
Epiglottic cartilage	Mucous covered, leaf-shaped anterior border of the laryngeal inlet	• Inferior aspect attached to thyroid by **thyroepiglottic ligament** • Anterior aspect attached to hyoid by **hypoepiglottic ligament**

Arytenoid cartilages (2)	• 3 sided, pyramidal-shaped:
	  1. Apex
	  2. Vocal process
	  3. Muscular process
	• Articulate with cricoid cartilage at **cricoarytenoid joints**
		• Apex: articulates with corniculate cartilages and is embedded within the aryepiglottic fold
		• Vocal process: posterior attachment for vocal ligament
		• Muscular process: attachment for lateral and posterior cricoarytenoid muscles

Corniculate cartilages (2)	• Articulate with apex of arytenoid cartilages • Embedded within aryepiglottic fold	Provide structure to aryepiglottic folds
Cuneiform cartilages (2)	Embedded within aryepiglottic fold	

(continued)

Skeleton of the larynx *(continued)*

Structure	Description	Significance
Thyrohyoid membrane	Attaches thyroid cartilage to hyoid	• Midline thickening is **median thyrohyoid ligament** • Lateral thickenings form **lateral thyrohyoid ligaments**
Vocal ligament	Extend from laryngeal prominence anteriorly to vocal process of arytenoid cartilages posteriorly	• Thickened, free superior border of conus elasticus • Covered by mucosa to form **vocal fold**
Quadrangular membrane	Extends from arytenoid cartilages to sides of epiglottic cartilages	• Free inferior border—**vestibular ligament,** covered by mucosa to form **vestibular fold** • Free superior border—**aryepiglottic ligament,** covered by mucosa to form **aryepiglottic fold**
Conus elasticus	• Superior border—vocal ligaments • Lateral extensions—**lateral cricothyroid ligaments**	• Continuous anteriorly with median cricothyroid ligament • Close tracheal inlet when vocal ligaments are approximated
Joints		
Cricothyroid	Articulation between inferior horns of thyroid and cricoid cartilage	Movements: rotation and gliding of thyroid on the cricoid
Cricoarytenoid	Articulation between arytenoid cartilages and cricoid cartilage	Movements: sliding of arytenoid cartilages—toward or away from each other, tilting and rotation of arytenoids

Clinical Significance

Fracture

Laryngeal fractures are common. They may produce hemorrhage and edema, obstruction of the airway, and hoarseness.

Muscles of the larynx

The extrinsic muscles of the larynx include the supra- and infrahyoid musculature described with the muscles of the neck and are involved in moving the larynx as a whole—suprahyoids elevate the larynx; infrahyoids depress the larynx.

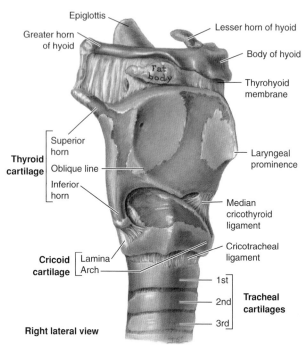

FIGURE 8-5. Skeleton of larynx, right lateral view. (From Moore KL, Dalley AF. *Clinically Oriented Anatomy.* 5th ed. Baltimore: Lippincott Williams & Wilkins; 2006:1090.)

The intrinsic muscles of the larynx move the skeleton of the larynx to alter tension on the vocal folds and the size of the rima glottidis.

Muscle	Proximal Attachment	Distal Attachment	Innervation	Main Actions
Vocalis	Arytenoid cartilage	Vocal ligament	Inferior laryngeal	Alter tension on vocal ligament for whispering
Cricothyroid	Cricoid cartilage	Thyroid cartilage	External laryngeal	Tenses vocal ligament

(continued)

Muscles of the larynx *(continued)*

Muscle	Proximal Attachment	Distal Attachment	Innervation	Main Actions
Thyroary- tenoid	Thyroid cartilage	Arytenoid cartilage	Inferior laryngeal	Relaxes vocal ligament
Lateral cricoary- tenoid	Cricoid cartilage			Adducts vocal folds
Posterior cricoary tenoid				Abducts vocal folds
Transverse and oblique arytenoids	Arytenoid cartilage	Contralateral arytenoid cartilage		Alter tension on vocal ligament

Additional Concept

Innervation

All intrinsic laryngeal musculature is innervated by branches of CN X. The external and internal laryngeal nerves are branches of the superior laryngeal nerve, which is a branch of CN X. The internal laryngeal nerves supplies sensory innervation superior to the vocal folds, whereas the external laryngeal nerves supplies the cricothyroid muscle. Sensory innervation inferior to the vocal folds and all of the remaining intrinsic musculature is supplied by the recurrent laryngeal nerve, via the inferior laryngeal branch.

ALIMENTARY STRUCTURES IN THE NECK

Pharynx and esophagus
(Figure 8-1)

The pharynx is the fibromuscular tube that serves as a common route for air and ingested substances. It extends from the base of the cranium to the inferior border of the cricoid cartilage of the larynx. It is divided into three parts based on what region/structure it lies posterior to and communicates with: (1) nasopharynx, (2) oropharynx, and (3) laryngopharynx. The esophagus, presented in the thorax chapter (see Chapter 1), extends from the pharyngoesophageal junction to its termination in the abdomen at the cardial orifice of the stomach. It is composed of voluntary, skeletal muscle in its upper third, a mixture of skeletal and smooth muscle in its middle third, and involuntary, smooth muscle as its inferior third. The innervation mirrors the musculature—the superior half receives somatic motor and sensory innervation, whereas the inferior half receives autonomic (vagal parasympathetic and sympathetic) and visceral sensory innervation.

Structure	Description	Significance
Nasopharynx	• Posterior to nasal cavity • Extends inferiorly to level of soft palate • **Pharyngeal tonsils**—located on posterior wall • **Auditory tube**—opens on posterolateral wall • **Salpingopharyngeal fold**—extends from torus tubaris to blends with pharyngeal muscles	• Communicates with nasal cavity via posterior choanae • Pharyngeal tonsils—aggregate of lymphatic tissue • Auditory tube (pharyngotympanic tube)—opening surrounded by cartilaginous torus tubaris and lymphatic elements—the **tubal tonsil** • **Salpingopharyngeus** underlies the mucosal that forms the fold; its contraction opens the auditory tube during swallowing
Oropharynx	• Posterior to oral cavity • Between soft palate and epiglottis • **Palatine tonsils**—located between palatoglossal and palatopharyngeal arches	• Receives bolus of food from oral cavity during swallowing • Palatine tonsils (tonsils)—aggregate of lymphatic tissue that lie in the **tonsillar bed:** formed by the superior constrictor and **pharyngobasilar fascia**—that fascia that fills space between the superior constrictor and the cranium
Laryngopharynx	• Posterior to larynx • Between epiglottis and cricoid cartilage • Communicates anteriorly with larynx at laryngeal inlet	• Walls formed by middle and inferior constrictor, palatopharyngeus, and stylopharyngeus muscles • **Piriform recess**—depression on each side of laryngeal inlet between pharyngeal wall and aryepiglottic fold

Additional Concept

Swallowing

Swallowing has three phases:

1. Stage 1: voluntary; food is formed into bolus and pushed into oropharynx
2. Stage 2: involuntary; soft palate elevates, pharynx widens and shortens
3. Stage 3: involuntary; pharyngeal constrictors force food inferiorly into esophagus

Blood Supply to the Pharynx

The longitudinally oriented pharynx receives branches from a host of arteries throughout its course, including tonsillar, ascending and descending palatine, lingual, and ascending pharyngeal arteries. Venous drainage parallels arterial supply.

Clinical Significance

Piriform Fossa

The superior laryngeal artery and internal and inferior laryngeal nerves lie just deep to the mucosa of the piriform fossa and are subject to damage when ingested objects become lodged here.

Muscles of the pharynx
(Figures 8-3 and 8-6)

The muscles of the pharynx are arranged into an external circular layer and an internal longitudinal layer. All laryngeal muscles are voluntary.

Muscle	Proximal Attachment	Distal Attachment	Innervation	Main Actions
External				
Superior constrictor	Pterygomandi-bular raphe, mandible, tongue, pterygoid hamulus	Pharyngeal tubercle of occipital bone and pharyngeal raphe	Pharyngeal plexus	Constricts pharynx
Middle constrictor	Stylohyoid ligament and hyoid bone	Pharyngeal raphe		
Inferior constrictor	Thyroid and cricoid cartilage			

(continued)

Muscles of the pharynx *(continued)*

Muscle	Proximal Attachment	Distal Attachment	Innervation	Main Actions
Internal				
Palato-pharyngeus	Palatine aponeurosis	Pharynx	Pharyngeal plexus	Tenses soft palate, elevates pharynx
Stylo-pharyngeus	Styloid process of temporal bone		CN IX	Elevates pharynx
Salpingo-pharyngeus	Torus tubaris of auditory tube		Pharyngeal plexus	

Additional Concept

Fascia of the Pharynx

The fascia covering the internal aspect of the pharyngeal constrictors is **pharyngobasilar fascia**, whereas the fascia on their external surface is **buccopharyngeal fascia**. The pharyngobasilar fascia combines with the buccopharyngeal

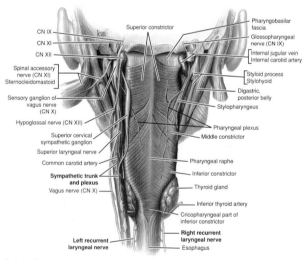

Posterior view

FIGURE 8-6. Pharynx and cranial nerves, posterior view. (From Moore KL, Dalley AF. *Clinically Oriented Anatomy.* 5th ed. Baltimore: Lippincott Williams & Wilkins; 2006:1105.)

fascia superior to the superior constrictor to fill the gap between the superior constrictor and the cranium.

Innervation

The musculature of the pharynx, with the exception of the stylopharyngeus, is supplied by the **pharyngeal plexus**. Motor fibers in the pharyngeal plexus are from CN X, whereas sensory fibers are from CN IX. The superior-most part of the nasopharynx receives sensory innervation from V_2.

Constrictor Muscles

The constrictors are arranged like a stack of nested flower pots, with gaps between each. The gaps allow structures to enter and leave the pharynx. The four gaps between:

1. superior constrictor and cranium—conveys levator palati, auditory tube, and ascending palatine artery
2. superior and middle constrictors—conveys stylopharyngeus, stylohyoid ligament, and the glossopharyngeal nerve
3. middle and inferior constrictors—conveys internal laryngeal nerve and superior laryngeal artery
4. inferior constrictor and esophagus—conveys recurrent laryngeal nerve and inferior laryngeal artery; the recurrent laryngeal nerve changes names to the inferior laryngeal nerve upon entering the larynx.

List of Mnemonics